An A–Z of Gynaecology

AN A–Z OF GYNAECOLOGY
with comments on aspects
of management and nursing

MARY ANDERSON
MB, ChB, FRCOG

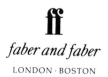

faber and faber

LONDON · BOSTON

First published in 1986
by Faber and Faber Limited
3 Queen Square London WC1N 3AU

Filmset by
Wilmaset Birkenhead Wirral
Printed in Great Britain by
Redwood Burn Limited
Trowbridge Wiltshire
All rights reserved

British Library Cataloguing in Publication Data

Anderson, Mary M.
An A–Z of gynaecology: with comments on aspects
of management and nursing.
1. Gynaecology
I. Title
618.1   RG101
ISBN 0–571–13966–3

Library of Congress Cataloging-in-Publication Data

Anderson, Mary M.
  An A–Z of gynaecology.
  Bibliography: p.
  Includes index.
  1. Gynecology—Handbooks, manuals, etc.
2. Gynecology—Practice—Handbooks, manuals, etc.
3. Gynecologic nursing—Handbooks, manuals, etc.
I. Title.
RG110.A53 1986   618.1   86-2119
ISBN 0–571–13966–3 (pbk.)

Contents

Preface

An 'A–Z' implies a completeness which this reference book cannot claim. Nevertheless, most gynaecological topics are mentioned with greatest stress on common clinical conditions. The subjects are discussed in alphabetical order for easy reference.

It is to be hoped that the book will prove useful not only to nurses but also to physiotherapists, social workers, health visitors and others working in areas where gynaecological problems may arise.

Acknowledgements

I am grateful to Mrs A. Evans, nursing officer, and Sister A. Henry, gynaecological ward sister, of Lewisham Hospital who have produced the nursing notes for this book. Their willing help, in spite of busy commitments, was greatly appreciated.

My thanks are due to Miss P. Downie, Medical Editor, whose guidance and encouragement are undoubtedly the driving force behind any such publication.

My thanks also to Mrs A. Besterman for help with the illustrations.

Figure 4/4 is taken from *Herpes, AIDS and Other Sexually Transmitted Diseases* by Derek Llewellyn-Jones, and is reproduced by permission of the publishers, Faber and Faber.

1. Anatomy and Physiology

A knowledge of basic anatomy and physiology is essential for the study of any aspect of medicine and none more so than gynaecology. The outline which follows is in no sense comprehensive but it is meant to serve as a useful reference. Larger textbooks of anatomy and physiology should be referred to for greater detail and suggestions for further reading are given at the end of this book.

Anatomy

Vulva

This word refers to the female external genitalia (Fig. 1/1) which consist of:

(a) *Mons pubis*. A pad of fatty tissue situated in front of the symphysis pubis covered by skin and hair.

(b) *Labia majora* (the 'large lips'). The two rounded folds of fatty tissue and skin extending from the mons above to the perineum below. Their outer surfaces are covered by hair. They are the female equivalent of the male scrotum.

(c) *Labia minora* (the 'small lips'). These lie within the labia majora, are smaller and more delicate than the labia majora. They are not covered by hair and contain many blood vessels and nerve endings. Superiorly, they split to enclose the *clitoris* and inferiorly they join at the *fourchette* or posterior border of the entrance to the vagina (the *introitus*).

(d) *The clitoris*. This is the female equivalent of the male penis and is a small sensitive erectile structure situated in the midline between the two folds of the labia minora. It is about 2.5cm long, the terminal 0.5cm being called the *glans*. It has a central corpus with two crura which are attached to the inferior pubic rami.

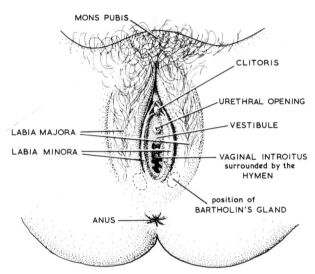

Fig. 1/1 The female external genitalia

(e) *The vestibule*. This is the area enclosed by the labia minora and into it opens the urethra above and the vagina below.

(f) *The vaginal introitus*. This opens on to the lower part of the vestibule. Before puberty and in virgins it is covered by an incomplete membrane known as the *hymen*. This is ruptured at the time of intercourse and further torn during childbirth when it is represented by tags of skin known as *carunculae myrtiformes*.

(g) *The perineum*. This is the area bounded by the vaginal fourchette anteriorly and the anus posteriorly.

The deeper structures of the vulva consist of (Fig. 1/2):

(a) *Vestibular bulbs*. These are two small collections of vascular erectile tissue lying on either side of the vaginal opening deep to the labia majora and minora. They are surrounded by the *bulbocavernosus muscles*. These muscles extend anteriorly to the clitoris and join the *ischiocavernosus* muscles which lie under the inferior pubic rami covering the crura of the clitoris.

(b) The *superficial* and *deep transverse perineal muscles* and the muscle forming the *external anal sphincter* join together with the posterior portion of the bulbocavernosus muscle to form the *perineal body*.

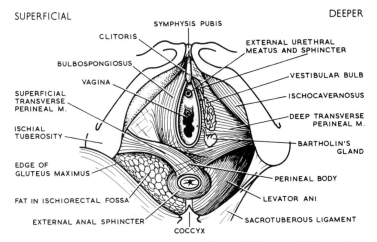

SUPERFICIAL

DEEPER

SYMPHYSIS PUBIS

CLITORIS

EXTERNAL URETHRAL
MEATUS AND SPHINCTER

BULBOSPONGIOSUS

VESTIBULAR BULB

VAGINA

SUPERFICIAL
TRANSVERSE
PERINEAL M.

ISCHOCAVERNOSUS

ISCHIAL
TUBEROSITY

DEEP TRANSVERSE
PERINEAL M.

EDGE OF
GLUTEUS MAXIMUS

BARTHOLIN'S
GLAND

PERINEAL BODY

FAT IN ISCHIORECTAL FOSSA

LEVATOR ANI

EXTERNAL ANAL SPHINCTER

SACROTUBEROUS LIGAMENT

COCCYX

Fig. 1/2 The deeper structures of the vulva, and the superficial muscles
of the pelvic floor

(c) *Bartholin's glands.* These lie one on either side of the posterior
part of the vaginal opening behind the vestibular bulbs and deep
to the labia. They secrete mucus thereby keeping the genitalia
lubricated.

(d) Deep to the vestibular and Bartholin's glands is a triangular area
bound by the transverse perineal muscles behind and the two
inferior pubic rami in front and on each side. In this area is the
urogenital diaphragm or *triangular ligament* (Fig. 1/3). Above it
are the deeper muscles consisting of the *compressor urethrae* in
front and the deep *transverse perineal muscles* behind.

(e) Posteriorly, in the space behind the transverse perineal muscles
is the *ischiorectal fossa* which is composed of fibro-fatty tissue.

Blood supply: This is from the internal iliac artery via the internal
pudendal vessels.

Nerve supply: This is mainly by the *pudendal nerve* which runs
forwards in the ischiorectal fossa to divide into posterior labial,
clitoral and other branches serving the vulval structures. Other
nerves supplying the vulva are the *ileo-inguinal nerve* anteriorly, and
a branch of the *sciatic nerve* posteriorly.

Lymphatic drainage: There is a rich supply of lymphatics and a

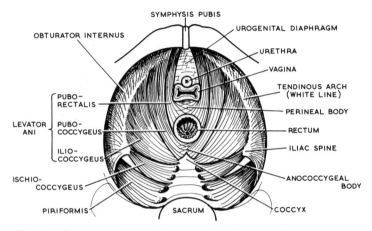

Fig. 1/3 The urogenital diaphragm and the levator ani muscles

knowledge of their drainage is of especial importance in dealing with carcinoma of the vulva.

There are four main groups of lymph nodes: the *superficial and deep inguinal* and the *superficial and deep femoral*. These in turn will drain into the deeper *iliac* and *obturator* lymph nodes.

Vagina (Fig. 1/4)

The vagina is an elastic fibromuscular tube leading from the vulva to the uterus. Its anterior wall is 8–10cm long, the posterior wall 12–14cm. At rest, the walls lie in close contact.

Its upper end is attached to the cervix which projects into it, and the recesses of the vagina thus formed are called the *fornices* (fornix, singular) of the vagina (anterior, posterior and two lateral).

STRUCTURE

The walls are composed of stratified squamous epithelium thrown up into numerous folds or *rugae*. This gives the vagina its elastic property so that it can stretch to accommodate the male penis and more particularly to allow the passage of the fetal head during childbirth.

Deep to the epithelium are:

(a) a layer of elastic vascular connective tissue,

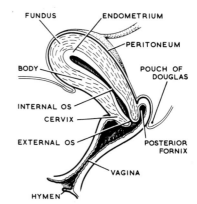

Fig. 1/4 A coronal view of the cervix and vagina

(b) a layer of involuntary muscle fibres arranged in a criss-cross manner, and

(c) an encircling layer of connective tissue containing blood vessels, lymphatics and nerves.

Passing down the anterolateral walls are the vestigial Wolffian or mesonephric ducts (Gartner ducts).

The pH of the vagina is acid – about 4.5 – due to the presence of lactic acid produced by bacterial action on glycogen from the squamous cells. These bacteria are called Döderlein's bacilli and the resulting acidity acts as a protector to the vagina preventing infection.

RELATIONS OF THE VAGINA (Fig. 1/5)

Anterior. The bladder and urethra.

Posterior. The perineal body, anus and rectum (from below upwards).

Lateral. (a) *Upper two-thirds* to pelvic fascia. The two ureters pass close to the lateral fornices.

(b) *Lower third*, muscles (levator ani, bulbocavernosus) and the vestibular bulbs (Bartholin's glands).

Superior. The uterus and cervix.

Inferior. The hymen and the vulva.

Blood supply: Branches from the internal iliac artery; uterine, vesical, middle rectal and internal pudendal arteries.

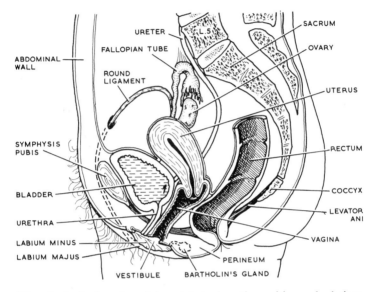

Fig. 1/5 Sagittal section of the pelvis to show the position and relations of the vagina, uterus and Fallopian tubes

Nerve supply: This is both sympathetic and autonomic.
Lymphatic drainage: Of the lowest third to the horizontal, to inguinal groups along with those from the vulva; of the upper two-thirds, to the internal iliac and sacral nodes.

Uterus (Fig. 1/6) (see also Fig. 1/4)
This is a hollow flattened pear-shaped organ lying in the true pelvis above the vagina. It measures 7.5 × 5 × 2.5cm and the cavity is 5–6cm in the adult.

It consists of two portions: the cervix or neck, and the body.

(a) *The cervix*: It is 2–3cm in length, and has a vaginal and a supravaginal portion. Its cavity is the cervical canal which communicates below with the vagina via the external os and above with the internal cavity via the internal os. It is lined by columnar epithelium.

It is attached to the pelvic walls by ligaments – the pubocervical anteriorly, the uterosacral posteriorly and the

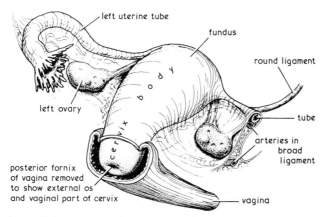

Fig. 1/6 Postero-lateral view of
the uterus, left Fallopian tube
and ovary

Fig. 1/7 The ligaments of the
cervix

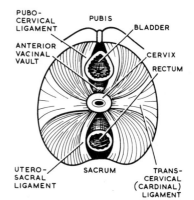

transverse cervical (cardinal or Mackenrodt's ligament) laterally
(Fig. 1/7). It therefore acts as a 'stabiliser' for the uterus.

(b) *The body*: The two Fallopian tubes are inserted into its upper
and outer angles. Above this, the area of the uterus is referred to
as the *fundus*. The *cornua* are the portions into which the tubes
are inserted. The *isthmus* is the narrower lower zone of the
uterus lying above the internal os.

STRUCTURE

1. The specialised lining of the body is called the *endometrium*.
2. The muscular walls of the uterus are the *myometrium* consisting

of several layers of interlacing smooth muscle fibres surrounding the blood vessels.

3. The *pelvic peritoneum* covers the uterus apart from the isthmus (see p. 23).

The normal position of the uterus is one of anteversion (rotated forward) and anteflexion (bent forwards on itself).

Blood supply: This is from the uterine arteries which arise from the internal iliac arteries.

Lymphatic drainage: (a) *The body*. To the pelvic nodes but also to the para-aortic nodes. Occasionally, spread may occur along the round ligament vessels to the inguinal nodes. (b) *The cervix*. To the obturator, the internal and the external iliac groups of nodes.

Nerve supply: This is from the sympathetic and parasympathetic systems.

RELATIONS (Fig. 1/5)

Anterior. The bladder and the uterovesical pouch of peritoneum with coils of intestines.

Posterior. The peritoneal cavity.

Lateral. The broad ligaments, Fallopian tubes, ovaries and round ligaments. Ureters lateral to cervix, crossed above by the uterine vessels.

Superior. The intestines.

Inferior. The vagina.

The Fallopian tubes (oviducts) (Fig. 1/8)

Lying one on either side of the uterus being inserted into the cornua, they are about 10cm long. They pass laterally towards the pelvic wall where they turn backwards and downwards to hang over the ovaries.

They have four distinct portions:

1. The *interstitial* part, the narrowest, lying within the uterine wall.

2. The *isthmus* extending for about 2.5cm laterally from the uterine wall.

3. The *ampulla*, the wider portion extending from the isthmus for about 5cm towards the lateral pelvic wall.

4. The *infundibulum*, the most lateral 2.5cm part, composed of numerous finger-like processes, the fimbriae, which surround

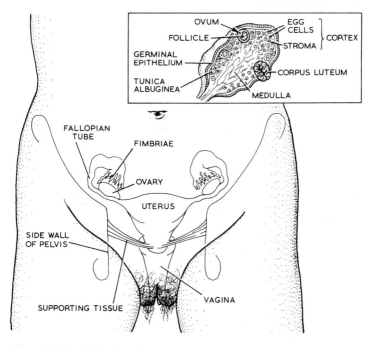

Fig. 1/8 The Fallopian tubes and ovaries. The inset drawing shows the structure of an ovary

the tubal opening. One longer fimbria is usually attached to the ovary.

STRUCTURE

1. Lining of cubical epithelium is thrown into folds or plicae. Most of the cells are ciliated (having hairs on them) so as to waft the ovum along on its journey from the ovary to the uterine cavity.
2. Vascular layer of connective tissue under the mucous membrane.
3. Inner circular layers of smooth muscle.
4. Outer longitudinal layer of smooth muscle.
5. Outer covering of peritoneum.

Blood supply: From the uterine and ovarian vessels.

Lymphatic drainage: Along with ovarian lymphatics to the aortic nodes.
Nerve supply: From the ovarian plexus.

RELATIONS (Fig. 1/5)
Medial. The uterus.
Lateral. The infundibulo-pelvic ligaments and lateral pelvic walls.
Anterior, superior and posterior. The peritoneal cavity and intestines.
Inferior. The broad ligaments and ovaries.

The ovaries (Fig. 1/8)
During maturity these are two almond shaped bodies, whitish in colour and corrugated in appearance measuring about 3 × 2 × 1 cm. They are attached to the posterior layer of the broad ligament by a mesentery called the mesovarium. They are suspended from the uterine cornua by the ovarian ligaments and laterally by the infundibulo-pelvic ligaments to the side walls of the pelvis.

STRUCTURE
1. The *medulla* is the inner part and is composed of loose connective tissue and blood vessels.
2. The *cortex* is the outer functional portion containing the follicles in various stages of development. Its outer fibrous covering is called the *tunica albuginea*.
3. A modified form of the peritoneum referred to as the *germinal epithelium* covers the ovaries.

Blood supply: The ovarian vessels from the aorta pass to the ovary via the infundibulo-pelvic ligaments.
Lymphatic drainage: To the aortic nodes.
Nerve supply: The ovarian plexus.

RELATIONS
Medial.   The body of the uterus and the ovarian ligaments.
Lateral.   The infundibulo-pelvic ligaments and the side walls of pelvis.
Anterior.   The mesovarium and the broad ligaments.
Posterior.   The peritoneal cavity and the intestines.

The peritoneum (Fig. 1/9)

Because the uterus, tubes and ovaries are placed transversely across the pelvis between the bladder and the rectum, the peritoneum lining the anterior abdominal wall extends down over the top of the bladder on to the anterior surface of the uterus (not the isthmus which therefore lies under a loose fold of peritoneum), over the

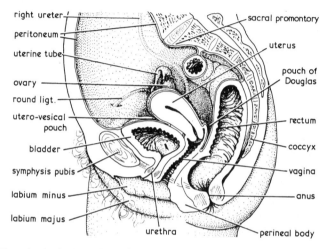

right ureter — sacral promontory
peritoneum —
uterine tube — uterus
ovary — pouch of Douglas
round ligt. —
utero-vesical pouch — rectum
bladder — coccyx
symphysis pubis — vagina
labium minus — anus
labium majus —
urethra — perineal body

Fig. 1/9 Sagittal section of the pelvis showing the peritoneum in the pelvis

fundus and down the posterior surface as far as the junction of the upper and middle thirds of the posterior wall of the vagina. It then covers the rectum and up over the posterior abdominal wall. Laterally, the peritoneum rises up to cover the tubes, descending behind them so that two folds are formed called the *broad ligaments*.

The pouch of peritoneum between bladder and uterus is called the *uterovesical pouch*; the pouch between uterus and rectum, the *pouch of Douglas*, its lateral margins being the *uterosacral folds* or ligaments.

The broad ligament fold contains the following structures: the Fallopian (uterine) tubes in its upper border, the ovarian ligaments, the round ligaments, and the ureters (on its base close to the vaginal fornices).

The pelvic floor muscles and the pelvic ligaments (see Figs. 1/3, 1/7)
The pelvic floor or diaphragm is formed by the various parts of the levator ani muscles. These are two strong muscles lying on either side of the pelvis arising from the pelvic walls and converging towards the midline to be inserted into the perineal body, the anal canal, the coccyx and the lower end of the sacrum. They are concave above and convex below forming therefore a muscular hammock across the pelvis.

There are three components:
1. The *pubococcygeus* arising from the back of the pubic bones to converge on the perineal body.
2. The *iliococcygeus* arises from the obturator internus fascia and sweeps downwards and inwards to be inserted into the ano-coccygeal body and the coccyx.
3. The *ischiococcygeus* arises from the spine of the ischium and passes downwards and inwards to be inserted into the coccyx and lowest piece of the sacrum.

It will be seen from Figure 1/3 that the urethra, the rectum and the vagina all pass through the pelvic muscles which therefore provide support for these organs.

The superficial muscles have already been mentioned (p. 14).

PELVIC LIGAMENTS

The *cervical ligaments* have also been mentioned (p. 18) and are the anterior pubocervical ligaments, the posterior uterosacral ligaments and the lateral cardinal or Mackenrodt's ligaments (Fig. 1/7).

The *round ligaments* pass from the cornua of the uterus forward and laterally in the broad ligament towards the internal inguinal rings through which they enter the inguinal canals to emerge through the external abdominal rings and be inserted in the fatty tissue of the upper end of the labia majora. They play only a small part in supporting the uterus.

The other ligaments have already been described but scarcely merit the title of ligament as they play little or no supporting role. These are the broad ligaments, the uterosacral ligaments, the ovarian ligaments and the infundibulo-pelvic ligaments.

The transverse cervical ligaments already described do anchor the cervix and therefore play a part in stabilising the uterus.

Physiology of Menstruation

This is the basic physiology which concerns us in gynaecology involving the ovaries and the uterus and the endocrine glands which control events.

Reproductive life begins at the menarche with the first period and ends with the cessation of menstruation at the menopause.

A summary of the events which occur during a menstrual cycle is shown in Table 1/1 and Figure 1/10.

Table 1/1   A summary of the stages of the menstrual cycle

		No. of days
1.	After menstruation a follicle ripens: oestrogen is produced: the endometrium proliferates	10
2.	Ovulation	
3.	The corpus luteum appears: progesterone is produced: small amounts of oestrogen persist: the endometrium becomes secretory	14
4.	The corpus luteum degenerates: oestrogen and progesterone levels fall: menstruation	4
	TOTAL	28

The endometrium

By the fifth day or so after menstruation, the endometrium shows proliferation of its glands and stroma. About the twelfth day the glands are greatly dilated and become secretory, the stromal cells swell and the capillaries form sinuses. Towards the end of a 28-day cycle the stroma becomes very vascular and oedematous, small haemorrhages and thrombi appear and finally the superficial layers of this thickened endometrium break down and are discharged as the menstrual flow.

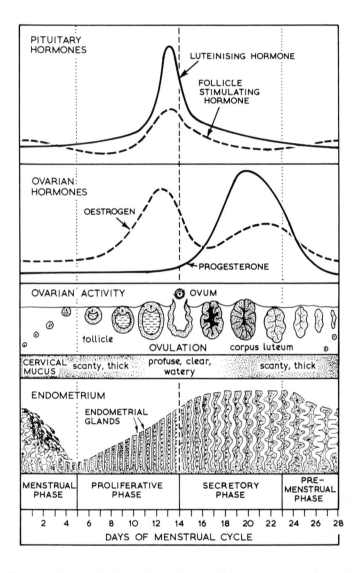

Fig. 1/10 Schematic description of the physiology of menstruation and ovulation

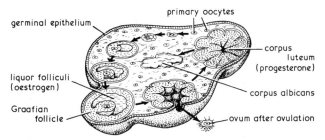

Fig. 1/11 The ovarian cycle

The ovary

It is the events in the ovarian cycle which produce these changes in the endometrium (Fig. 1/11).

The cortex of the ovary contains the primordial follicles or 'egg cells'. At birth the ovary contains some 200 000 of these but only comparatively few will mature. They are known as *Graafian follicles*.

During the first part of an ovarian cycle some follicles ripen and come to the surface of the ovary. One of these reaches the surface first, ruptures and releases the egg or ovum. Ovulation has occurred and takes place about the fourteenth day of a 28-day cycle. The empty follicle collapses in on itself and during the second half of a cycle a yellowish-red structure forms called the corpus luteum.

The ovary releases hormones during its cycle:
1. Oestrogen from the developing follicle
2. Progesterone from the corpus luteum.

Hypothalamic-pituitary cycle (Fig. 1/12)

The above series of events is controlled by what happens at the level of the hypothalamus and the pituitary gland.

From the hypothalamus are produced 'releasing' factors called gonadotrophin releasing hormones (GnRH). These stimulate the anterior pituitary to release two hormones called follicle stimulating hormone (FSH) and luteinising hormone (LH) into the circulation. The cerebral cortex itself may, it should be noted, influence the activity of the hypothalamus.

The follicle stimulating hormone (FSH) stimulates a few sensitive follicles in the ovary to mature and from these oestrogen is produced.

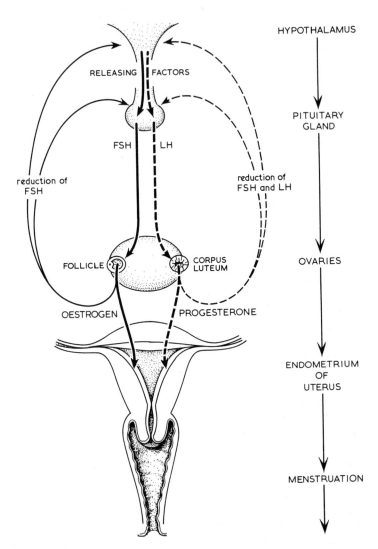

Fig. 1/12 The control of menstruation

The rising level of oestrogen has a negative 'feedback' effect on the secretion of FSH and only the larger follicles continue to grow.

These larger follicles go on producing oestrogen which, when it reaches a sufficiently high level, has a positive feedback effect causing a surge in the production of FSH and LH but mainly LH, and it is this surge which causes ovulation.

The corpus luteum formed after ovulation produces progesterone and this added to the circulating oestrogen seems to exert a negative feedback effect on the pituitary so that levels of both FSH and LH fall.

Unless fertilisation and implantation of the ovum occur the corpus luteum degenerates, oestrogen and progesterone levels fall and can no longer support the endometrium which has thickened throughout the cycle as described. It then breaks down and is discarded as menstruation.

As the corpus luteum degenerates, the negative feedback mechanism fails and the hypothalamus produces gonadotrophin releasing hormone again, thereby initiating a new cycle.

2. Benign Disorders

Abortion

The correct medical term for a miscarriage. It means the ending of a pregnancy before viability of the fetus which is normally before 28 weeks or under 1.5kg in weight. Abortion is classified into the following types.

THREATENED ABORTION
There is some bleeding but no pain and the pregnancy continues.

INEVITABLE ABORTION
There is bleeding with pain and dilatation of the cervix. The pregnancy will ultimately abort.

INCOMPLETE ABORTION
Part of the pregnancy has been expelled but portions remain and bleeding continues.

MISSED ABORTION
The ovum dies but the uterus retains it instead of expelling it. Spontaneous expulsion may ultimately occur but, usually, it is realised clinically that the pregnancy is not progressing (usually by ultrasound scanning) and arrangements are then made to empty the uterus by curettage or by extra-uterine prostaglandin if the size of the uterus is greater than about 12 weeks.

THERAPEUTIC ABORTION
This is more usually termed 'termination of pregnancy'. Under the provisions of the Abortion Act 1967, a pregnancy may be

terminated taking various physical, mental and social factors into account. Two registered medical practitioners must consider the case and two signatures are required on the legal document. The operation is carried out vaginally by either suction curettage or, abdominally (if too far advanced for the vaginal approach), by the instillation of prostaglandins or by the operation of hysterotomy. With the increasing use of prostaglandins this latter operation, which is in effect a 'mini' caesarean section, is rarely carried out nowadays.

SEPTIC ABORTION
Any of the above abortions which become infected will be described as a 'septic abortion'. Emptying of the uterus and giving antibiotics (having sent high vaginal swabs to the laboratory for culture) will control the sepsis.

HABITUAL ABORTION
Where more than three spontaneous abortions occur. If they are early abortions, before 14 weeks, a genetic or endocrine cause may be likely, although it is usually impossible to demonstrate either of these. Late abortion may be due to the so-called incompetent cervix where the internal os region of the cervix is lax and allows a pregnancy of over 14 weeks to protrude through it and so ultimately abort.

Management of abortion
This depends on the type of abortion as assessed by the history and examination. In summary:
1. *Threatened abortion*: Treated by bed rest (not necessarily in hospital) until all signs of bleeding have ceased. Thereafter mobilisation of the patient can be allowed but sexual intercourse should be avoided until the pregnancy is obviously continuing satisfactorily.
2. *Inevitable and incomplete abortion*: Here hospitalisation is necessary because of the risk of haemorrhage. Evacuation of the uterus by curettage (usually suction curettage which is safer). Blood transfusions may be necessary in some cases. *It is important to remember that anti-D antigen should be given to Rhesus-negative women.*
3. *Habitual abortion*: Investigation of this problem will include:

- x-ray hysterography to assess the shape of the uterine cavity and exclude a developmental abnormality;
- chromosome studies on the blood of both husband and wife; and
- general examination of the patient including assessment of her thyroid and renal functions.

Nursing notes

THREATENED ABORTION
1. Bed rest will need to be supervised.
2. The urine should be tested daily for protein.
3. Any vaginal loss should be carefully observed.
4. Reassurance should be given to the patient and her partner.

INCOMPLETE ABORTION
1. Postoperative observations not only of the blood pressure and pulse but also of any vaginal loss.
2. Adequate analgesia should be given, according to the doctor's directions.
3. Counselling should be given to the patient and her partner.
4. Information and advice concerning local support groups should be offered.

LATE THERAPEUTIC ABORTION
At all times the patient should be kept informed regarding the proposed procedure, such as an intravenous infusion. The nurse should be involved in the total care of the patient during all stages of a late therapeutic abortion. In particular she should:
1. Supervise modified bed rest.
2. Allow fluids only.
3. Make half-hourly observations of the blood pressure and pulse.
4. Monitor pain, and note the start of contractions.
5. Regulate the infusion rate according to instructions.
6. Give analgesia as required.
7. Attend the patient during delivery of the fetus.
8. Inform the doctor on delivery of the fetus.
9. Dispose of the products of conception according to local practice (they may be required for laboratory testing).

The patient may wish to have her partner with her during the procedure. She may also wish to see the fetus.

Following delivery of the fetus the nurse should:
1. Carefully observe temperature; respiration rate and pulse; blood pressure; and note any vaginal loss.
2. Support emotionally the patient, her partner and any other member of the family who may be distressed.
3. Arrange referral for counselling as necessary.

Adenomyosis

A form of endometriosis in which the endometrial glands and stroma invade the myometrium of the uterus. It may form a tumour-like area but without a capsule and this is called an *adenomyoma*.
Symptoms and signs: Usually found in older infertile women; the uterus tends to be enlarged and painful periods develop which are heavier than normal.
Diagnosis can only finally be made after removal of the uterus and examination of it by the pathologist.
Treatment may be conservative as for endometriosis (see p. 47) or surgical by removal of the uterus.

Adrenogenital syndrome

A better descriptive name is *congenital adrenal hyperplasia*. The condition is due to a group of enzyme defects which prevent the synthesis of cortisone. Adrenocorticotrophic hormone (ACTH) is produced in quantity causing hyperplasia of the adrenal gland and the production of excess androgens.

Three different forms of the syndrome are seen, the most severe involving sodium loss; unless detected in the infant, death results. Cortisone must be given to sustain life. Cases detected late in life present with virilisation.

Amenorrhoea

Literally, 'without menstruation'. Lack of menstruation is physiological before the onset of periods – the menarche – and after cessation of periods – the menopause. Amenorrhoea may be primary or secondary.

Primary amenorrhoea: Where no menstruation has previously occurred. The menarche usually takes place between the ages of 10 to 16. Investigations for failure to menstruate will be initiated after the age of 16.

Secondary amenorrhoea: Failure to menstruate after a period of normal menstruation.

Most causes of amenorrhoea can apply to either type.

Pregnancy
This must always be considered in every age-group, whatever the patient says.

Psychological stress
(a) Amenorrhoea is common in young girls under particular social or emotional stress, e.g. leaving school, beginning a new job, boyfriend problems, rows at home, and so on.
(b) Dietary: Excessive and too rapid loss of weight may result in amenorrhoea. Anorexia nervosa is an extreme example.

Endocrine disorders
Thyroid disease may result in cessation of periods.

Adrenal diseases such as hyperplasia or Cushing's disease may also be associated with amenorrhoea.

Ovarian disease such as polycystic ovaries or premature ovarian failure will result in amenorrhoea. Physiological ovarian failure occurs at the time of the menopause – before that the term *premature ovarian failure* is used.

Hyperprolactinaemia is a condition where there is an excessive amount of circulating prolactin – a hormone from the anterior pituitary. This inhibits the production of FSH and LH with resulting amenorrhoea. Hyperprolactinaemia is due to a pituitary tumour (an adenoma or micro-adenoma) or it may be associated with drugs such as phenothiazine or methyldopa. The circulating prolactin level is physiologically raised during lactation after childbirth.

Developmental abnormalities

1. Chromosomal abnormalities such as Turner's syndrome or testicular feminisation will be associated with amenorrhoea (primary).
2. Vaginal or uterine abnormalities may present with amenorrhoea. One such is *cryptomenorrhoea* where the menstrual flow is built up behind a closed hymen – an imperforate hymen – and may present as a lower abdominal swelling accompanied by pain.

Other associations with amenorrhoea are systemic diseases of any severity, e.g. glandular fever and tuberculosis, or the use of the contraceptive pill which may result in temporary secondary amenorrhoea when it is discontinued.

INVESTIGATIONS

History: including	– primary or secondary
	– exposure to pregnancy
	– recent drugs
	– recent illness
	– weight loss or gain
	– stress.
Examination	– development (or lack) of secondary sexual characteristics, such as the breasts, body hair, etc
	– imperforate hymen
	– enlargement, e.g. uterus (pregnancy).
Special tests: including	– x-rays of chest and pituitary fossa
	– measurements of hormones (FSH, LH, oestrogen, progesterone, prolactin)
	– laparoscopy to view the pelvic organs and take biopsies of the ovaries if indicated.

TREATMENT

This is of the cause, for example:

Psychological stress: Explanation is often sufficient.

Dietary causes: Dietary advice and supervision.

Thyroid and adrenal diseases: Appropriate control.

Hyperprolactinaemia: Treatment with the drug bromocriptine. Surgery or radiotherapy for some pituitary tumours may be necessary.

Imperforate hymen: Surgical incision of the imperforate hymenal membrane and drainage of the old menstrual blood.

Polycystic ovaries and post-pill amenorrhoea: These causes may be amenable to the drug clomiphene citrate used to induce ovulation. It is used where not only menstruation but pregnancy is desired.

Anovulation

'Without ovulation'. Whereas normal menstrual cycles include ovulation, that is the production of an egg or ovum about mid-cycle, not all cycles are accompanied by ovulation. These are then known as anovulatory cycles. Such cycles are often irregular and the bleeding may be heavy and prolonged or short and scanty – *dysfunctional uterine bleeding*.

The presenting symptom may be irregular or abnormal menstruation or it may be infertility. The diagnosis may be made by recording the basal temperature which fails to show the normal biphasic change of the ovulatory cycle, or, more certainly, by sampling the endometrium in the second half of the cycle. In a normal ovulatory cycle the endometrium would show secretory changes; in an anovulatory cycle the endometrium remains proliferative in appearance. Measurement of the serum progesterone on or about day 21 of the cycle will also be diagnostic.

Of itself anovulation does not matter but in problems of infertility induction of ovulation is important. This may be achieved by giving the drug clomiphene citrate or if this fails a combination of FSH and LH obtained from an extract of human menopausal gonadotrophin – Pergonal. This is followed by human chorionic gonadotrophin to provide the LH 'surge'. This latter regime must, however, be used under strict laboratory control.

Apareunia

This means inability to have intercourse. In the male this usually means impotence, for which there are many causes which must be investigated by a specialist.

In the female, apareunia may be due to *organic disease*, for example, an unduly thick hymen, vulval scarring (after childbirth), acute inflammatory conditions; or there may be *psychological causes*.

This is the commonest reason and results in vaginismus or spasm of the vaginal sphincter muscles.

After excluding a physical cause the patient may be helped by psycho-sexual counselling when fear or ignorance may be recognised and removed. More profound psychological disturbances may require the help of a psychiatrist.

Arrhenoblastoma

This is a rare tumour of the ovary forming less than 1 per cent of all ovarian tumours. It produces male sex hormones which result in masculinisation of the female. In 20 per cent the tumour is malignant.

Artificial insemination

Where a husband lacks spermatozoa or where he is impotent and unable to inseminate his wife, spermatozoa may be injected directly into the uterine cavity at the time of ovulation with the aim of achieving fertilisation.

The injected specimen may be that of the husband – artificial insemination from the husband (AIH) or it may be from a donor (AID).

Asherman's syndrome

A rare condition where intra-uterine adhesions are formed following excessive curettage, usually for late postpartum bleeding. The diagnosis can be made by a hysterogram (instillation of radio-opaque material into the uterine cavity) or by an ultrascan. Treatment is unsatisfactory but gentle curettage to break down adhesions may be successful, or, more recently, insertion of an intra-uterine device has been used.

Bartholinitis

Acute inflammation of Bartholin's gland and its duct is occasionally seen and may be due to gonococcal infection. More usually an infection presents as a Bartholin's abscess. There is a tender tense swelling in the region of Bartholin's gland on one side. Treatment is to drain the abscess, usually under general anaesthesia. This is done mostly by the procedure of *marsupialisation* which involves excising an oval of skin and abscess wall and suturing skin and abscess wall together to create an open pouch for continuing drainage.

A *Bartholin's cyst* may develop in the gland or duct and is best excised or 'marsupialised' since it is prone to infection and abscess formation.

Nursing care

Following excision of a Bartholin's cyst the nurse should:

1. Carry out the standard observations following an anaesthetic.
2. Remove the pack or wick on the first postoperative day.
3. Encourage the patient to take a bath twice a day to promote healing.
4. Teach the patient vulval toilet.

Breakthrough bleeding

A term which implies bleeding between periods in someone who is on the contraceptive pill. Usually only spotting, it can nevertheless be quite heavy. If it persists and is troublesome, a change of pill giving a higher dosage of the progestogen component is usually sufficient to stop it.

Brenner tumour

This is a rare tumour of the ovary usually found in older age-groups. It is solid, composed of fibrous and epithelial elements and forms about 2 per cent of all solid ovarian tumours.

Candidiasis

Infection of the vagina with the fungus *Candida albicans* – monilia or thrush – is common. It may occur in association with a concurrent illness, especially if antibiotics are being taken. It may also arise in diabetics or during pregnancy, and there appears to be a higher incidence in women on the contraceptive pill.

The *symptoms* are of vulval and vaginal irritation and soreness. On examination there is a thick curdlike discharge. Swab culture will confirm the diagnosis.

Treatment is by one of the several antifungal agents now available. The commonest is nystatin given in the form of vaginal pessaries, with nystatin cream for skin irritation.

Cervicitis

Literally, inflammation of the cervix. Acute inflammation may be caused by gonorrhoea and is associated with a purulent discharge and a congested inflamed cervix. More commonly seen is chronic cervicitis with or without an erosion (see p. 51). There is excess mucopurulent discharge, and enlarged follicles on the cervix may be seen.

Treatment is by cautery using either electrocautery or cryocautery – the application of frozen carbon dioxide gas. The resulting dead tissue sloughs off over a period of time and is replaced by fresh covering tissue.

Chlamydia

See sexually transmitted diseases, page 75.

Chocolate cyst

Strictly speaking, this term refers to an ovarian cyst into which bleeding has occurred and that blood has become inspissated into thick tarry altered blood. This can happen to any type of ovarian cyst which has bled but, by usage, the term tends to refer to the cysts seen in association with endometriosis (see p. 47).

Climacteric

The word used to refer to the period of time leading up to and immediately following the cessation of periods – the menopause. This period of time is often referred to as the menopause or more colloquially as 'the change'. The time involved varies from one to five years or more and a variety of symptoms may be experienced. These will be described under *menopause*, page 62.

Cryptomenorrhoea

Literally 'hidden menstruation'. During normal development the hymen, which is a thin fold of tissue lined by squamous epithelium lying over the vaginal orifice, breaks down to form an incomplete membrane. If it remains closed, however, it acts as an obstruction to the flow of menstrual blood, which builds up behind it to fill first the vagina (haematocolpos), then the uterine cavity (haematometra) and finally the tubes (haematosalpinx). The condition is also known as *imperforate hymen*.

The *diagnosis* is usually made by examination of a girl complaining of primary amenorrhoea over the age of 16 and frequently with cyclical symptoms of lower abdominal pain. On examination a lower abdominal swelling may be found and on separating the labia the distended hymen may be seen, bluish in colour because of the altered blood behind it.

Treatment is to make a cruciate incision into the hymen under general anaesthesia and to drain the blood. Trimming of the thickened hymen may also be necessary.

Cushing's syndrome

Not, strictly speaking, a gynaecological condition, it may nevertheless be diagnosed by the gynaecologist during investigations for, for example, amenorrhoea.

The basic pathology is overactivity of the adrenal gland in association with a tumour (basophil adenoma) of the anterior pituitary gland.

The syndrome consists of a 'moon face' appearance, obesity, hirsutism, hypertension and often associated diabetes. A similar picture may result with prolonged use of cortisone. Plasma cortisol levels are used to make the diagnosis.

Cystadenoma

See ovarian tumours, page 64.

Cystocele

A bulging downwards of the anterior wall of the vagina carrying the bladder with it. See prolapse, page 71.

Decubital ulcer

In complete prolapse (third degree, or procidentia) the uterus and cervix appear outside the vulva. The epithelium covering the exposed cervix and uterus becomes whitened and thickened (keratinised) but is prone to disturbance of circulation and actual ulceration may occur. These ulcers are known as decubital ulcers and if present may delay surgery until they are healed. This is achieved by reducing the prolapse and maintaining the reduction if necessary by packing, thereby improving the epithelial circulation and allowing healing of the ulceration to occur.

Nursing care
1. Daily vaginal douching by the insertion of a flavine vaginal pack. Oestrogen cream may be prescribed for use before packing.
2. A well-balanced diet should be encouraged.
3. A regular soft bowel action should be ensured.

Dermoid cyst

See ovarian tumours, page 64.

Discharge

The commonest discharge met with in gynaecology is the *vaginal discharge*. There are no actively secreting glands in the vagina so in a sense the term is a misnomer. Nevertheless the glands of the cervix produce a discharge as does the normal 'wear and tear' on the vaginal epithelium.

Some discharge is normal and physiological. It becomes pathological when it is excessive or infected, causing discomfort or irritation.

Leucorrhoea is a word sometimes used to describe an excessive amount of normal discharge – a difficult thing to assess since it varies with the fastidiousness of the patient.

A discharge arising from infection is associated with a *vaginitis* – an inflammation of the vagina. There are three main types:
1. Monilial vaginitis (or candidiasis) (see p. 38).
2. Trichomoniasis vaginitis (see p. 79).
3. Non-specific bacterial vaginitis.

This last appears to be due to the normal bacteria of the vagina which for an unknown reason have become pathogenic. Culture and sensitivities may be possible, otherwise empirical treatment is given, such as an acid jelly (Acijel) or metronidazole or Sultrin cream.

In older women significant vaginal discharge may be due to inflammation of the vaginal skin secondary to its becoming thin and reddened – an effect of oestrogen lack. The use of local oestrogen cream is helpful in this situation.

Other causes of vaginal discharge are (a) a foreign body such as a retained tampon; (b) chemical due to douching or insertion of pessaries to which there is an allergy; and, of course, (c) malignant conditions of the vagina, cervix and uterus must never be forgotten.

Once diagnosed each requires treatment in its own right.

Dysfunctional uterine bleeding

A term which indicates abnormal menstruation not associated with pathology such as fibroids. It is due to an upset in oestrogen/progesterone levels for a reason that is unknown and it is one of the commonest gynaecological complaints.

There are different patterns of dysfunctional bleeding: excessive loss but normal cycle – menorrhagia; too frequent menstruation – epimenorrhoea; prolonged menstruation; and prolonged menstrual cycle. All these are usually accompanied by ovulation.

Anovulatory cycles (without ovulation) may give rise also to a variety of irregular bleeding among which is the so-called metropathia haemorrhagica or cystic glandular hyperplasia (see p. 62). Here there is a prolonged cycle with hyperplasia of the endometrium occurring because of excess oestrogen stimulus. When the oestrogen level falls, bleeding will follow which is prolonged and heavy.

The *diagnosis* of dysfunctional bleeding is made by (a) the clinical history and (b) excluding pathology such as fibroids or carcinoma of the endometrium (a D and C may be carried out).

Treatment will depend on the severity of the condition and the age of the patient.

1. Full discussion, reassurance and explanation with, perhaps, an iron supplement may suffice in milder forms. Psychological factors frequently play a large part in dysfunctional bleeding.
2. Oestrogen/progestogen preparations such as the contraceptive

pill will help younger patients.

3. Progestogen alone, such as norethisterone, given for 7–10 days premenstrually will control the cycle.
4. Anti-fibrinolytic agents such as epsiaminocaproic acid have been used with some success.
5. Anti-prostaglandins such as indomethacin (Indocid) may help in cases of menorrhagia, as may the drug danazol.
6. In older women with resistant dysfunctional bleeding where anaemia may be a problem, hysterectomy may well be the best solution.

Dysmenorrhoea

Painful periods. This may be either *primary* dysmenorrhoea (from virtually the onset of menstruation) or *secondary* dysmenorrhoea (developing after years of comfortable menstruation).

The basic pathology of menstrual pain is not understood, although it is realised that many factors are involved. It is the case that anovulatory cycles are painless.

The *management of primary dysmenorrhoea* is therefore either pain relief by using, for example, paracetamol, or by using anti-prostaglandins such as mefenamic acid (Ponstan), (prostaglandin produces increased uterine muscle activity with some ischaemia and therefore pain); or by creating anovulatory cycles by the use of the contraceptive pill. If the girl also needs a contraceptive this last is the ideal treatment for her. Progestogen alone may be of value.

In secondary dysmenorrhoea organic disease must be looked for. Two main conditions are endometriosis and pelvic inflammatory disease. By treating these appropriately the pain will be alleviated.

Although frequently thought of as largely psychological, dys-menorrhoea *is* a very real entity which gives rise to a lot of distress and days off work, school or college. It therefore warrants careful assessment, exclusion of associated disease and adequate treatment.

Dyspareunia

Pain during sexual intercourse. The pain may be *superficial* (at the introitus or vaginal entrance) or *deep* (in the pelvis or lower abdomen). There is a variety of causes.

Superficial:
1. Painful scarring, e.g. episiotomy.
2. Acute vulvitis or vaginitis due to infection.
3. Enlargement or infection of a Bartholin's gland.
4. Atrophy and shrinkage of the skin around the introitus seen in some postmenopausal women.
5. Congenital abnormalities such as a septum across the lower vagina.

Deep:
1. Endometriosis involving especially the uterosacral ligaments.
2. A retroverted uterus with ovaries prolapsed in the pouch of Douglas where pressure on even normal ovaries causes pain.
3. Chronic pelvic infection.

Vaginismus (see p. 79) is an involuntary contraction of the pelvic floor muscles which in itself will produce pain. While it may occur as a 'protective' mechanism in association with any of the above causes of pain it frequently results from fear or apprehension or dislike of coitus.

In the *management* of dyspareunia, therefore, a careful clinical history must be obtained and a gentle pelvic examination carried out to try to establish the cause. Other investigations may include laparoscopy to obtain a direct view of the pelvic organs.

Treatment is of the cause and where no organic lesion is detected psycho-sexual counselling may be required.

Dysplasia

This means partial loss of structural and functional resemblance to the parent tissue. Thus we talk of cervical dysplasia where changes are seen in the cervical cells ranging from mild dysplasia with normal cytoplasm but large irregular nuclei, to severe dysplasia with irregularity of the cells also. This verges on carcinoma.

The term used is *cervical intra-epithelial neoplasia* (CIN) and the grades are:
CIN I   – mild dysplasia
CIN II – moderate dysplasia
CIN III – marked dysplasia and carcinoma.

Dystrophy

The definition of this word is 'a disorder of the structure and function of an organ or tissue'. Usually congenital, e.g. muscular dystrophy. In gynaecology it is used as for the vulval dystrophies, leucoplakia and kraurosis.

Ectopic pregnancy (Fig. 2/1)

A pregnancy occurring in a site other than in the uterine cavity. The commonest site is in the Fallopian tube but pregnancies have been described in an ovary and in the abdominal cavity.

FALLOPIAN TUBE

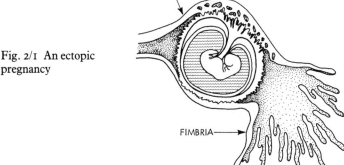

Fig. 2/1 An ectopic pregnancy

FIMBRIA

The *cause* of an ectopic pregnancy is unknown but there is an association with tubes damaged by infection (which reduces their motility and therefore ability to transfer the fertilised egg down to the endometrial cavity). The incidence of tubal pregnancies is also higher in the presence of an intra-uterine device.

The *outcome* of a tubal pregnancy may be either to abort from the fimbrial end of the tube into the pelvic cavity with some slow blood loss which may collect in the pouch of Douglas to form a pelvic haematocele; or to rupture through the wall of the tube with much more severe haemorrhage and collapse of the patient.

Signs and symptoms
1. A period may be missed giving the possibility of a pregnancy, or the last period may have been abnormally light.

2. There is lower abdominal pain and if severe the patient may faint.
3. Abnormal vaginal bleeding or a dark discharge may occur.
4. Pelvic examination reveals considerable pelvic pain, and an important feature is exquisite pain produced by moving the cervix (due to the peritoneal irritation of blood lying in the pelvic cavity). This is called *cervical excitation pain*.
5. In cases of rupture and severe haemorrhage the patient becomes shocked rapidly.

Diagnosis
In addition to the above features the diagnosis may be made by:
1. Ultrasound scan: Not however entirely reliable.
2. Laparoscopy.
3. A standard immunological pregnancy test is positive in 75 per cent of cases and is not therefore specific. To measure the beta sub-unit of HCG is more accurate if facilities are available.
4. Laparotomy: If the case seems certain clinically then laparotomy should be proceeded to forthwith. In the case of a collapsed patient with a ruptured ectopic, laparotomy should be carried out without delay so that the bleeding vessels may be clamped and the haemorrhage stopped.

Management
The damaged tube is removed. Rarely, the pregnancy can be shelled out and the tube repaired. The ovary on the side of the ectopic is not removed.

Unfortunately there is a higher risk in such a case of a subsequent ectopic – presumably due to the fact that tubal damage was already present to some extent on the other side.

Nursing care
Following laparotomy for an ectopic pregnancy the nurse should:
1. Carry out standard postoperative observations including the regular recording of the blood pressure and pulse and careful observation of any vaginal loss.
2. Supervise the intravenous infusions of blood/other fluids.
3. Administer analgesia as required.
4. Note any wound drainage and remove the drain when the drainage becomes minimal.

5. Ensure the patient's comfort by carrying out all nursing procedures necessary.

Nothing is allowed by mouth until bowel sounds have returned. Once this has occurred small amounts of clear fluids are allowed, progressing to a light diet.

1st postoperative day: Gentle mobilisation may start. Chest physiotherapy and leg exercises should be given, and encouraged by the nurses.

2nd postoperative day: Glycerine suppositories (2) should be given (if necessary) to relieve flatus.

3rd postoperative day: The wound dressing should be removed and left exposed.

5th postoperative day: If clips have been used, they should be removed.

6th postoperative day: Sutures should be removed.

Throughout the postoperative period the patient and her partner should be given support and reassurance. Before leaving the hospital they should be referred for counselling as necessary.

Endometriosis

A condition in which pockets of endometrial tissue grow outside the endometrial cavity. Its aetiology is unknown.

The areas of ectopic endometrium may develop within the muscle wall of the uterus. This is internal endometriosis or *adenomyosis* (see p. 33). External endometriosis mainly occurs in the pelvis with deposits of black-coloured 'spots' visible on the uterosacral ligaments, the uterovesical fold of peritoneum, the floor of the pelvis and on the ovaries. Cysts may form in the ovaries which are filled with inspissated blood – the so-called chocolate cysts (see. p. 39). These may be small or large and the ovary becomes adherent to surrounding structures, quite dense adhesions often developing.

Endometriosis may be found in more distant sites, the explanation for some of which is difficult to understand. For example, deposits may be found in the umbilicus, caecum, appendix, round ligament, laparotomy scar (especially if surgery has involved opening the uterine cavity, such as at hysterotomy, myomectomy or caesarean section).

Theories of aetiology

1. Retrograde spill of menstrual blood back through the tubes and into the pelvic cavity.
2. Conversion of primitive cells into endometrial tissue, 'cell metaplasia'.
3. Cells carried by lymphatics or via the bloodstream, that is an embolism.

There are probably several factors involved.

Symptoms and signs

Typically the patient is in her late twenties or thirties, nulliparous and often infertile. She experiences pain prior to her periods and, if pelvic endometriosis exists, deep dyspareunia (pain on intercourse) (see p. 44) occurs. On examination the pelvic organs are often felt to be 'fixed' – by adhesions. Tenderness over the ovaries and uterosacral ligaments with a feeling of irregularity – 'knobbliness' – over the uterosacral ligaments may be noticeable. Large cysts may be present.

In adenomyosis the uterus is bulky and tender.

Diagnosis

The clinical history and findings may be suggestive, but to be certain lararoscopy should be carried out and the pelvis inspected directly. Spots of endometriosis look like little black pin heads – 'pheasants' eyes' they are referred to – but if the pelvis is simply stuck down by adhesion the diagnosis may be difficult to differentiate from old pelvic inflammatory disease. If biopsy is possible then the histological appearances of endometrial cells will confirm the diagnosis.

Treatment

MEDICAL

Hormone therapy is useful. In younger patients the *contraceptive pill* may be used but *progestogens* alone are better. These are given continuously or cyclically, e.g. norethisterone 5mg twice daily from day 15 to day 25 of the cycle.

The drug of choice is *danazol* which inhibits the pituitary gonadotrophins and is therefore anti-oestrogenic (see p. 113).

SURGICAL

This is indicated in the older woman with severe symptoms and widespread involvement of her pelvic organs. Total abdominal hysterectomy and bilateral salpingo-oophorectomy is carried out and hormone replacement therapy may be given afterwards to relieve any menopausal symptoms.

Endometritis

This is a condition which is often not identified clinically but is, rather, a histological diagnosis. As its name suggests it is an inflammation of the endometrium. It may follow childbirth, abortion or the insertion of an intra-uterine contraceptive device. In its acute phase it presents as a pelvic infection with pain, discharge, fever and systemic upset.

Chronic endometritis is rare simply because the endometrium sheds itself at regular intervals. There are no symptoms and the diagnosis will be made histologically. A long-standing intra-uterine contraceptive device may be associated with chronic inflammatory changes in the endometrium and tuberculosis is also a well-known but fairly rare cause of chronic endometritis.

Senile endometritis is infection arising in the postmenopausal endometrium – usually in the elderly. Damming back of pus can occur because of stenosis of the cervix (sometimes by tumour) and the uterine cavity fills with pus. This is known as *pyometra*.

Malignancy of the endometrium must always be excluded at the curettage which accompanies the dilatation of the cervix (done to drain the pus).

Endotoxic shock

In some cases of septicaemia a state of shock may develop with circulatory failure. At first, the body's response is a pyrexia and vasodilatation with a rapid pulse. Mild hypotension may be noted at this stage. When circulatory failure ensues there are pallor, cold extremities, a thready almost imperceptible pulse and increasing loss of consciousness. Untreated endotoxic shock will lead to renal failure, brain damage and death.

CAUSAL ORGANISMS IN GYNAECOLOGY
Anaerobic streptococci; coliform bacillus; *Clostridium welchii*.

PRECEDING CONDITIONS
Incomplete abortion; criminal (self-procured) abortion; pelvic infection.

Management
Urgent skilled treatment is required and the patient is best nursed in an intensive care unit. In brief:

1. *Treat the infection*
   Having taken swabs for bacteriological examination commence broad spectrum antibiotics.
   If pus is located in the pelvis or elsewhere surgical drainage may be indicated.

2. *Improve the circulation*
   Intravenous fluids are necessary and plasma expanders, such as dextran, may be indicated.
   If the clotting mechanism is affected, fresh blood or plasma is given.
   If respiratory distress ensues, ventilation of the lungs may be necessary.
   If the heart is affected, digitalisation and other cardiac supportive drugs may be required.
   If renal failure ensues, dialysis will be required.
   If vasoconstriction is marked and unresponsive to adequate transfusion, then vasodilators will be given.

The management, both medical and nursing, of such cases is highly skilled and details are beyond the scope of this book.

Enterocele

Seen on clinical examination as a 'bulge' of the upper part of the posterior vaginal wall it consists of the peritoneum of the pouch of Douglas protruding downwards through the uterosacral ligaments carrying small bowel or even omentum in it. It is usually part of a prolapse but may occur in isolation, especially after hysterectomy. It is a true hernia and its treatment is surgical, namely to open the sac, excise it and close it with suturing of the uterosacral ligaments together under it to act as support.

Epimenorrhoea and Epimenorrhagia

These words are derived from the Greek and mean respectively frequent menstruation and frequent heavy menstruation. For causes see under dysfunctional uterine bleeding, page 42.

The use of Greek-derived words such as these is traditional in gynaecology but can be confusing and it is better to say exactly what you mean, e.g. frequent periods which are heavy.

Erosion

The normal cervix is covered by smooth squamous epithelium – skin, in other words. Under certain circumstances this may recede from the external cervical os leaving a well-defined area round the os which looks red and granular and may bleed to the touch. This is known as a cervical erosion. It may be associated with excess discharge because of the exposure of the cervical glands, and chronic cervicitis may be superimposed.

Cervical erosions may be congenital, they may follow childbirth or abortion, or result from infection.

Treatment

If there are no symptoms treatment is not necessary. If symptoms such as discharge or contact bleeding are present then treatment is indicated. Cauterising the erosion will destroy the unhealthy tissue and as healing occurs squamous epithelium grows in to cover the area. Cautery may be done by *electrocautery* – this usually requires a general anaesthetic – or by *cryocautery* which means the application of frozen carbon dioxide gas (see p. 94) – this procedure does not require a general anaesthetic.

Fibroids (Fig. 2/2)

These are benign tumours of the muscle wall of the uterus and are the commonest tumours found in women. They consist of unstriped muscle fibres supported by fibrous tissue. They are most commonly found in older women (over 35 years of age) who have not had children or are of low parity. An exception to this rule is African and West Indian women who have a higher incidence of fibroids in young and parous women. The aetiology of fibroids is unknown.

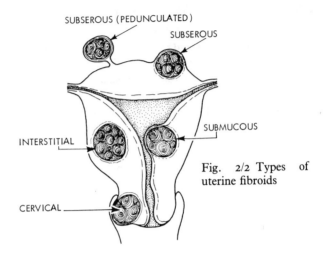

Fig. 2/2 Types of uterine fibroids

Sites

1. Within the wall of the uterus – *intramural* (interstitial).
2. Just under the peritoneal surface of the uterus – *subserous*.
3. Just under the endometrial surface – *submucous*.
4. With a long pedicle – on the uterine surface or within the cavity
   – a *pedunculated fibroid* and a *fibroid polyp*.
5. In the cervix – a cervical *fibroid*.
6. In the broad ligament – a *broad ligament fibroid*.

Signs and symptoms

1. If the fibroids are large and multiple the patient may be aware of a *lower abdominal swelling*.
2. *Bowel and bladder symptoms* (e.g. constipation and frequency of micturition) may occur because of pressure from the fibroid mass.
3. *Heavy menstruation* if the uterine cavity is enlarged by the fibroids.
4. Fibroids can undergo degeneration – cystic, hyaline, calcification. Torsion of a pedicle may occur. Red degeneration (necrobiosis) (see p. 75) with bleeding into, and softening of, the fibroid is found in association with pregnancy. All these may give rise to pain, especially the latter two. Malignant (sarcomatous) change is very rare.

Treatment

Only larger fibroids with symptoms need to be treated. Small ones can be ignored, especially near to the menopause, after which they will regress in size. The two methods of treatment are:

1. *Myomectomy*
   This means removal of the fibroids only, leaving the uterus. This is only suitable for younger women wishing to perserve their uterus and where relatively few fibroids are present.

2. *Hysterectomy*
   This is the treatment of choice for older women past the reproductive age-group.

Fistulae

A fistula is a pathological connection between structures and in gynaecology the commonest are between the uterus or vagina and the ureter, bladder or bowel.

The two most encountered are the *vesico-vaginal* fistula (bladder to vagina) and the *recto-vaginal* fistula (rectum to vagina).

They are infrequently seen in developed countries with good obstetric care and skilled gynaecological surgery; they are more common in underdeveloped countries where it is estimated that 85 per cent are due to obstructed labour.

Aetiology

1. Obstructed labour or traumatic delivery.
2. Trauma to ureter, bladder or bowel during surgery. Not common, but associated with pelvic surgery for cancer or endometriosis where dense adhesions exist.
3. Radiation for carcinoma may produce bladder or rectal fistulae (but rarely).

Symptoms

Incontinence of urine or faeces.

Investigations

The fistula will be demonstrated by, for example, instilling methylene blue dye into the bladder and placing swabs in the vagina. The upper swab will demonstrate ureteric fistula, the middle, bladder, and the lower, urethral. Intravenous urography, cystoscopy and sigmoidoscopy with barium studies of the bowel may be used in diagnosis.

Treatment
1. *Conservative*
   If recognised early many fistulae will heal spontaneously, e.g. bladder drainage by catheter for 2 to 3 weeks may allow a vesico-vaginal fistula to close.
2. *Surgical*
   Operation is required for most fistulae especially long-standing ones.

Galactorrhoea

Inappropriate lactation due to a high level of circulating prolactin – the hormone from the anterior pituitary which physiologically initiates and maintains lactation following childbirth.

The milky discharge from the nipples is usually associated with amenorrhoea. The cause is a high level of circulating prolactin and the source of this is a tumour of the anterior part of the pituitary gland – either a *macro*-adenoma or a *micro*-adenoma. The former is demonstrable by x-rays or scanning of the pituitary, the latter is not so demonstrated and is a presumed diagnosis. Certain drugs such as the contraceptive pill, phenothiazine derivatives and methyldopa may cause galactorrhoea.

The *diagnosis* is confirmed not only clinically but also by the laboratory measurement of high levels of prolactin in the blood.

The *treatment* is to give the drug bromocriptine which suppresses the level of prolactin. A detectable tumour of the pituitary will require surgical or radiotherapy treatment. Drug-induced galactor-rhoea should disappear on cessation of the drug concerned.

Gardnerella vaginalis

This organism may normally inhabit the vagina but as a Gram-negative low-grade pathogen it can be grown on culture of a vaginal swab taken from a woman complaining of discharge and found to have a vaginitis. Treatment is then required and the organism usually responds to a course of metronidazole.

Gonadal dysgenesis

A condition in which the ovaries fail to develop properly and therefore production of oestrogen is low or even absent. There are associated chromosome abnormalities. The secondary sexual characteristics fail to appear and the internal genitalia remain immature. These girls are sterile but can be helped to develop physically by the administration of oestrogens.

Gonorrhoea

See sexually transmitted diseases, page 76.

Gynaecomastia

Inappropriate enlargement of the breasts, as in men and in babies. In babies it is due to a spill-over of excess oestrogen from the mother which may remain active for a time in the circulation and in the female fetus may cause enlargement of the breasts. Occasionally vaginal bleeding may occur from the prematurely stimulated endometrium.

No treatment is required as the level of circulating oestrogen will subside in due course and these effects disappear.

Haematocele

A collection of blood in the pouch of Douglas. The usual cause is bleeding from a tubal pregnancy.

Haematocolpos

Distension of the vagina with blood.

Haematometra

Distension of the uterine cavity with blood

The above two conditions are most likely to arise when the introitus is closed by an imperforate hymen. See cryptomenorrhoea, page 40.

Haematosalpinx

A Fallopian tube distended with blood. The most common cause is a tubal pregnancy.

Herpes, genital

See sexually transmitted diseases, page 76.

Hirsutism

Excess hair, especially with a male distribution on the legs, arms, abdomen and face, is not uncommon among women. Because it can often cause embarrassment and distress among young women especially, help may be sought from the gynaecologist in the mistaken belief that it must be caused by some abnormality of hormone. It rarely is.

Causes
1. A familial or racial tendency.
2. Certain drugs such as phenytoin and steroids.
3. Adrenal disease.
4. In association with the polycystic ovary syndrome (see p. 68).
5. Idiopathic.
6. Functional.

(1) and (5) above are the most common causes. In idiopathic hirsutism a raised serum testosterone may be found, but it is often normal.

Treatment
1. Reassurance and explanation.
2. Electrolysis, waxing and other cosmetic devices.
3. The appropriate treatment for adrenal or ovarian disease.
4. Cyproterone acetate is an anti-androgen and is dramatically effective in some cases.

Hydrosalpinx

A Fallopian tube filled with clear fluid. When a tube is blocked at the fimbrial end the rest of the tube may fill up with secretions distending it and thinning out the walls, destroying the lining mucosa. It may be seen as part of a chronic pelvic inflammatory picture.

Hymen, imperforate

See cryptomenorrhoea, page 40.

Hyperprolactinaemia

A pathologically raised level of prolactin giving rise to galactorrhoea (see p. 54) and amenorrhoea (see p. 33).

Incontinence of urine

Urinary incontinence of one kind or another and to a greater or lesser extent is not uncommon in women.

Types

STRESS INCONTINENCE
When a sudden increase in intra-abdominal pressure, such as coughing or running, causes leakage of urine. This may be due to pelvic floor weakness or prolapse (see p. 70) or to instability of the bladder muscle (the detrusor).

URGENCY INCONTINENCE
When an irresistible desire to micturate occurs and, before a toilet can be reached, involuntary micturition occurs. Detrusor instability may be the cause, or infection, or even bladder carcinoma.

OVERFLOW INCONTINENCE
Where there is obstruction to normal urinary flow and dribbling from the overflow. Causes of obstruction are pelvic tumours such as fibroids or ovarian cysts.

NEUROLOGICAL INCONTINENCE
Incontinence in the old is caused by failure of nervous inhibition of

the detrusor muscle. Diseases such as multiple sclerosis may also be associated with urinary incontinence.

TRUE INCONTINENCE

Where there is a urinary fistula (see p. 53) incontinence of urine will occur.

Diagnosis

A careful history and clinical examination will often be sufficient to indicate which is the type of incontinence.

Bladder studies using cystometry and x-rays may be required. Other investigations are culture of the urine, intravenous pyelography, cystoscopy.

Treatment

This will depend on the cause, but may include:

1. Surgery for bladder and urethral prolapse and fistula.
2. The appropriate antibiotic where there is an infection.
3. Muscle-relaxant drugs to inhibit detrusor activity, e.g. propantheline bromide; emepronium bromide.
4. Physiotherapy to tone up pelvic floor muscles.
5. Oestrogens to improve the state of the lining mucosa of the bladder.
6. Various incontinence devices available for the elderly and those suffering from irreversible neurological disease.

Infertility

Failure to conceive. It may be *primary* (never having conceived) or *secondary* (a previous pregnancy having reached term or ending as a miscarriage).

Investigations for infertility are begun after one year of normal sexual activity. Eighty per cent of women trying to conceive are pregnant after one year.

The cause of infertility may lie with either the male or the female. Both should be investigated together.

The chief causes of infertility and their approximate incidence are shown below.

1. Defective ovulation   25%
   anovular cycles
   inadequate luteal phase
   oligomenorrhoea
   amenorrhoea
2. Defective semen   25%
   oligospermia
   azoospermia
3. Tubal blockage   15%
4. Other gynaecological abnormalities   7%
   fibroids
   endometriosis
5. Immunity problems   3%
   sperm antibodies
6. Normal couple – no abnormalities found   25%
7. Rare problems
   endometrial tuberculosis
   systemic disease
   non-consummation

Investigation of infertility is best shown in the form of a flow chart (Fig. 2/3, p. 60):

Treatment

Essentially, treatment of *female* infertility depends upon the cause, for example:

Failure to ovulate – drug therapy by clomiphene or Pergonal.

Hyperprolactinaemia – bromocriptine.

Blockage of tubes – surgery or in vitro fertilisation (the test tube baby).

The treatment of *male* infertility is unsatisfactory. Surgery may help where a varicocele is present. Hormone therapy does not seem to be particularly useful.

Intermenstrual bleeding

Bleeding between menstruation. It may range from slight spotting to quite heavy loss.

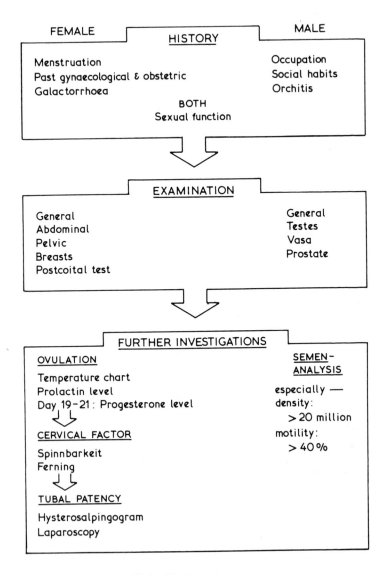

Fig. 2/3 Flow chart of infertility investigations

Causes
1. Mid-cycle bleeding associated with ovulation.
2. Contact bleeding due to a cervical lesion such as an erosion or a carcinoma.
3. 'Breakthrough' bleeding while on hormone therapy such as the contraceptive pill (see p. 38).
4. As part of dysfunctional uterine bleeding (see p. 42) in association with either prolongation or shortening of the luteal phase.

Diagnosis
Made by careful history taking, examination and cervical swab for cytology and possibly by a diagnostic D and C.

Kraurosis

A type of chronic epithelial dystrophy of the vulval skin. It is characterised by thinning and shrinkage of the skin and occurs in the elderly. It gives rise to pruritus and pain and responds usually to local oestrogen cream. It is *not* a pre-malignant condition.

Leiomyoma

The gynaecological term for this tumour of the uterus is *fibroid* or *fibromyoma*.

Leucorrhoea

An outdated word for vaginal discharge.

Leukoplakia

Another form of vulval skin dysplasia. It is characterised by irregular thickening and whitening of the skin in older women. It gives rise to pruritus and pain. It is a pre-cancerous condition and must be watched carefully, with biopsies if necessary. Symptoms may be relieved by steroid or oestrogen creams, but in intractable cases, or if suspicious cells are found on biopsy, excision of the vulval skin will be necessary.

Meig's syndrome

A rare condition consisting of ascites and hydrothorax in conjunction with a benign ovarian fibroma.

Menopause

Strictly speaking the cessation finally of menstruation. The word is more commonly used to refer to the years during which cessation of menstruation occurs. The correct word for this is 'climacteric'. Menstruation ceases most commonly between the ages of 45 and 55.

The menopause (or climacteric) may not be associated with untoward symptoms or signs but when they do occur tend to be of the following groups:
1. *Vasomotor.*   Hot flushes, palpitations, headaches.
2. *Metabolic.*   Vulval and vaginal skin changes (thinning, shrinkage); bladder mucosa thinning ('cystitis'); osteoporosis – thinning of bone structure.
3. *Psychological.*   Depression, irritability, insomnia.
Many symptoms met with at this stage of life are related to age itself or to the inevitable change in the 'life situation' at this age.

Treatment, if required, will be by understanding and supportive advice, hormone replacement therapy (a combination of small doses of oestrogens and progesterone) and occasionally by tranquillisers and antidepressants.

Menorrhagia

Heavy, but regular menstruation. It may be caused by fibroids or be part of a dysfunctional uterine bleeding picture due to hormone upset. *Diagnosis* is by history and examination; *treatment* is of the cause, e.g. D and C to examine the endometrium and give hormones accordingly; removal of fibroids (myomectomy) in younger patients wishing to retain the uterus; or hysterectomy in older women.

Metropathia haemorrhagica

An older term for what is now called cystic glandular hyperplasia. A form of dysfunctional uterine bleeding, it is due to too much oestrogen and too little progesterone acting on the endometrium. The patient suffers from prolonged, often heavy, menstruation. The endometrium when examined under the microscope shows many dilated non-secretory glands.

The *treatment* is either hormonal, by adding in a progestogen in the latter part of the cycle or by giving the combined 'pill', or in older women hysterectomy may be necessary.

Metrorrhagia

Irregular heavy menstruation. The causes are similar to menorrhagia. In older women cancer of the endometrium must be excluded by a diagnostic D and C.

Mittelschmerz

Pain occurring at mid-cycle and associated with ovulation.

Mole, hydatidiform

This abnormality of early pregnancy is rare in the UK occurring about 1 in 2000 pregnancies. There is no fetus and the trophoblast undergoes a degenerative change in which the villi become hydropic and appear clinically as masses of tiny grape-like structures.

Nowadays, the diagnosis is made because of greater use of ultrasound scanning, but the condition may be suspected because of certain clinical features:
1. The uterus is bigger than would be expected for the dates
2. Excessive nausea and vomiting are very common
3. No fetal heart can be detected with the sonicaid
4. Bleeding may occur.

The diagnosis used to be made by finding the standard urine test for pregnancy (based on urine output of HCG) being positive in high dilutions. Nowadays, ultrasound scanning will be used, if available.

The aetiology of the condition is unknown. Because of the risk of haemorrhage, perforation of the uterus from the invasive trophoblast and late development of malignancy (choriocarcinoma), when the diagnosis is made, the uterus *must* be emptied. This can be done by suction curettage. A repeat curettage is usually done a week or two later especially if irregular bleeding persists. Long-term follow-up of these cases is carried out at regular intervals for two years, the level of HCG being measured in 24-hour urine samples.

Moniliasis

See thrush infection, page 78.

Oligomenorrhoea

Infrequent periods. The aetiology is closely akin to that of secondary amenorrhoea (see p. 33).

Oophoritis

An inflammation of the ovary. This is unlikely to occur in isolation, and is most often seen as part of a bilateral inflammation of both tubes and ovaries.

Ovarian tumours

There is a wide variety of solid and cystic tumours of the ovary. For a detailed classification, one of the textbooks of gynaecology should be consulted (see Bibliography, p. 117).

A brief summary of the classification is:

1. *Non-neoplastic tumours*
   - follicular cysts arising from the follicles
   - luteal cysts arising from the corpus luteum
   - endometriotic cysts.

2. *Neoplastic tumours*
   (a) Epithelial
     - serous cyst (benign) (Fig. 2/4)
     - mucoserous cyst (benign)
     - endometrioid carcinoma (malignant)
     - Brenner tumour (rare, benign) (see p. 38)

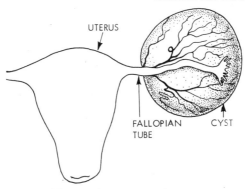

Fig. 2/4 A serous ovarian cyst

(b) Sex-cord tumours
   – granulosa cell tumour (low malignancy)
(c) Germ-cell tumours (from the oocytes)
   – teratoma or dermoid cysts (benign or, rarely, malignant)
(d) Connective tissue tumours
   – fibroma (both benign or malignant)
   – lipoma
(e) Metastatic tumours (from gastro-intestinal tract)
   A Krukenberg tumour of the ovary is usually secondary to a
   primary in the stomach.

Diagnosis of ovarian tumours
The important thing is to make a diagnosis as early as possible. An
ovarian swelling of over 7cm is considered to be suspicious and
laparotomy is indicated for its removal. Unfortunately, malignant
disease of the ovary tends to be 'silent' with few, if any, early
warning signs, so that when seen the patient may already have
extensive disease.

Symptoms
1. None. Found on routine pelvic examination.
2. Pressure symptoms (if large). Pelvic discomfort and even
   urinary retention may occur. Gastro-intestinal disturbance
   ('indigestion') is common in malignant tumours.
3. Pain, as a result of an accident to the cyst, e.g. torsion; haemorrhage into the tumour; rupture (especially cystic tumours).

4. Endocrine disturbances with upset of menstruation are rare except in 'functioning' tumours which produce hormones such as oestrogen.

Signs
Unless the patient presents as an emergency with acute symptoms of pain because of an accident to the tumour, the most usual sign is to find a swelling on examination either of the abdomen if the tumour is large enough to extend into the abdomen or on pelvic examination. If malignant change has occurred then associated signs may occur such as ascites.

Diagnosis
Ultrasound scanning has greatly advanced the ability to diagnose ovarian tumours and laparoscopy may also be valuable in doubtful cases. When the diagnosis is made laparotomy is mandatory.

Treatment
Surgical removal is the early treatment, and all tumours more than 7cm in diameter (some would say 5cm) must be removed as there is always the possibility of malignancy. In older women or where there is obvious malignancy, the uterus, cervix, tubes and both ovaries must be removed and in the case of clinical malignancy the omentum is also excised. This is because secondary deposits occur at an early stage in this site.

In young women removal of the cyst or tumour only will be carried out – an ovarian cystectomy. Further surgery will be required later if the tumour proves to be malignant.

FURTHER MANAGEMENT OF OVARIAN CARCINOMA
(see also p. 85)
As extensive surgery as possible is fundamental; even in apparently hopeless situations, with spread of tumour throughout the pelvic and/or abdominal cavity, as much of the tumour mass as possible should be removed. This is called *de-bulking* the tumour.

The mainstay of treatment thereafter is chemotherapy and at the time of writing cisplatinum and adriamycin are favoured and are often highly successful drugs.

Radiotherapy is of value when the growth has been apparently confined to the pelvis.

Pelvic inflammatory disease (PID)

PID can be acute or chronic and in the acute phase presents as a febrile illness accompanied by pelvic pain and signs of genital tract infection. It is synonymous with salpingitis or salpingo-oophoritis and is almost always bilateral. It is rare in women who are not sexually active.

Aetiological factors

1. Sexually transmitted infection, e.g. *N. gonorrhoea*.
2. Ascending infection by endogenous organisms, e.g. anaerobes.
3. Following D and C, termination of pregnancy, insertion of coil, etc.
4. Following a miscarriage or full time delivery.
5. Secondary spread of infection from, e.g. appendix.

At the present time PID constitutes a major problem and while several factors are involved there appears to be a direct relation to casual promiscuity among all age-groups, but young people in particular.

Outcome

The chronic picture is fairly typical.

1. Pelvic pain which is worse with menstruation and at the time of menstruation.
2. Heavy irregular menstruation.
3. Infertility. It has been estimated that acute PID results in infertility in 15 to 20 per cent of cases.
4. Ectopic pregnancy, as a result of permanent tubal damage.

Diagnosis

ACUTE PID

1. Acute onset of pelvic pain; vaginal discharge.
2. Pyrexia.
3. Raised WBC.
4. Tender appendages (tubes and ovaries) on vaginal examination. A pelvic mass (abscess) may be present.
5. Laparoscopy (if thought necessary) will reveal swollen reddened tubes with sero-purulent exudate.

Differential diagnosis is chiefly from appendicitis, ectopic pregnancy, or torsion or rupture of an ovarian cyst.

Treatment to be effective must be vigorous. Bacteriological swabs are taken from the upper vagina, cervix and urethra; also from the pelvic cavity if laparoscopy is being performed.

Broad spectrum antibiotics are given in combination with metronidazole. Intravenous fluids may be necessary in the ill patient and in these cases the antibiotics can be given intravenously in the first instance.

CHRONIC PID
This is difficult to treat and in fact is not curable by conservative measures.

Typical clinical features are heavy irregular and painful periods, dyspareunia and often infertility. The only condition which is similar in symptomatology is endometriosis (see p. 47).

Treatment
Courses of antibiotics and short-wave diathermy to the pelvis are measures which may provide relief for a time. Ultimately, in the more severe cases and even in younger women the uterus, tubes and ovaries may have to be removed.

Polycystic ovaries

As the name suggests this is a condition in which the ovaries contain multiple cystic follicles under a thickened smooth capsule. The older name for the condition is the Stein-Leventhal syndrome.

The clinical features are usually secondary amenorrhoea with infertility, and the patients are often (but not always) fat and hairy.

At laparoscopy (or they can be detected by ultrasound) the ovaries are found to be enlarged, smooth walled with a typical 'oyster' appearance. Ovarian biopsy will show the typical features. Hormone levels are not very helpful although the level of luteinising hormone may be raised as may the urinary 17 ketosteroids.

Treatment
Depends on the presenting problem.

1. *Obesity*. Diet.
2. *Infertility*. Ovulation is induced by clomiphene or tamoxifen.
3. *Oligomenorrhoea*. In itself this is immaterial but regular periods may be induced by clomiphene or tamoxifen. This renders the patient fertile, a fact that *must* be given to her.
4. *Wedge resection of the ovaries*. An operation in which a wedge of the ovaries is removed and as a result in many cases ovulation results. How the operation works is unclear and indeed is not used much nowadays since drug therapy is a successful alternative.

Polypus (or more commonly, polyp) of the cervix

This is a nodular or pedunculated (with a pedicle) growth arising from the endocervix and protruding as a red fleshy tag of tissue from the external os of the cervix. It is usually associated with cervicitis.

The polypus may be symptomless but may be associated with excess discharge, intermenstrual bleeding and postcoital bleeding.

Polyps should be avulsed, sent for histology (although malignancy is rare) and the base cauterised by diathermy or cryocautery.

Other forms are endometrial and fibroid polyps.

Postmenopausal bleeding

Any bleeding occurring from the genital tract one or more years after the last menstrual period.

All women who report postmenopausal bleeding must be investigated quickly by D and C to exclude endometrial carcinoma. Cervical carcinoma, which usually presents in younger age-groups anyway, is excluded by examination of the cervix, cervical smear and biopsy if necessary. Other causes of postmenopausal bleeding are atrophic vaginitis or, less commonly, vaginal infection.

All cases of postmenopausal bleeding must be regarded as being due to carcinoma until proved otherwise.

Premenstrual syndrome

Most women experience some form of discomfort in the week or 10 days prior to menstruation – lower abdominal aching, bloatedness, breast discomfort, irritability. In an exaggerated form this symptom complex has been given the title 'premenstrual syndrome'. The cause is unknown. Its features are:

1. Age about mid-thirties most commonly.
2. Marked tension, irritability, depression, headaches.
3. Abdominal swelling, breast tenderness, swelling of fingers and ankles.
4. It has been shown that accidents, suicides and criminal acts are more common in women at this phase of the cycle.

Treatment

Since the cause is unknown there is no standard method of treating the problem.

1. Sympathetic, interested listening and discussion are important.
2. Progestogen or progesterone can be given from mid-cycle.
3. High doses of vitamin B_6 have proved helpful in some cases.
4. Diuretics may be of some value.
5. Danazol in suppressive doses may be used in some severe cases.
6. Psychiatric help may, in rare instances, be required.

Prolapse

Literally, a 'slipping forwards'. The word implies a 'dropping' or herniation of one or more of the structures composing the genital tract through the pelvic diaphragm. It is due to the ligaments and muscles supporting the uterus and vagina becoming weakened and ineffective. Prolapse is common in older women who have had children and who are overweight. It may occur, however, in young nulliparous women.

Types of prolapse

UTERINE PROLAPSE (Fig. 2/5)
The uterus and cervix descend to varying degrees.

First degree.   The cervix descends to about half way down the vagina.

Second degree. The cervix appears at the introitus.

Third degree.   A complete prolapse where both uterus and cervix descend completely out of the vagina. Sometimes called *procidentia*.

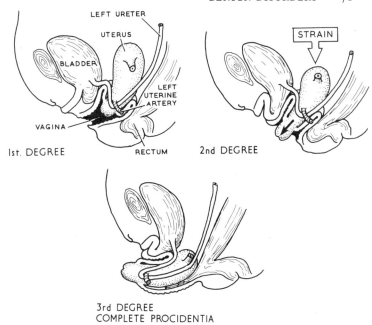

Fig. 2/5 Degrees of uterine prolapse

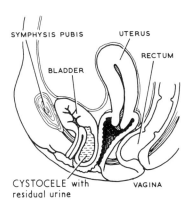

Fig. 2/6 A cystocele

CYSTOCELE (Fig. 2/6)
Bulging of the anterior wall of the vagina carrying the bladder base with it.

RECTOCELE
Bulging of the posterior wall of the vagina carrying the rectum with it.

ENTEROCELE
Herniation of the pouch of Douglas carrying a portion of the small bowel or omentum with it. It appears as a bulge behind the cervix at the top of the posterior wall of the vagina.

Clinical features of prolapse
These depend on the type of prolapse and its severity.
(a) The patient may complain of feeling 'something coming down' and may actually have felt or seen a lump appearing below the introitus.
(b) Urinary symptoms vary from frequency to actual difficulties with micturition relieved only by pushing back the prolapse. Stress or urge incontinence may or may not be associated.
(c) Difficulty with defaecation or a feeling of incomplete emptying of the bowel.

The *diagnosis* is made by careful examination asking the patient to cough and strain. The full extent of a prolapse may not, however, be assessed until the examination which is made under anaesthesia prior to surgery.

Complications of prolapse are rare. Ulceration of the exposed cervix may result in chronic neglected cases. These are called *decubitus ulcers* (see p. 41). Discharge and bleeding may occur and, rarely, malignant change.

In long-standing cases of cystocele, where bladder emptying is incomplete, chronic infection may develop with hypertrophy of the bladder wall, reflux and hydronephrosis. It must be stressed that these complications are rare.

Treatment
1. If prolapse is minimal with few symptoms no active treatment is required other than advice on measures to reduce weight, stop smoking and thereby improve a chronic cough, and so on.

2. Physiotherapy in the form of pelvic floor exercises may offer some help, but its main place is as a preventive measure following childbirth.

3. Surgery is the main form of treatment nowadays regardless of the age of the patient (see p. 101). Vaginal hysterectomy may be carried out with or without an anterior or posterior repair depending on whether a cystocele or rectocele is present. A Fothergill or Manchester repair in which the cervix is amputated and the cardinal ligaments thereby shortened may be the operation of choice although it has been largely superseded by vaginal hysterectomy. Where women wish to have more children it is best to defer surgery until childbearing is completed.

4. Pessaries, usually circular and made of plastic, are devices which can be used to support a prolapse. The posterior part of the ring fits into the pouch of Douglas, the anterior part rests against the pubic symphysis. There are other shapes of device but they are not in use nowadays. The pessary has the disadvantage of having to be changed at regular intervals otherwise it causes a smelly discharge and, if neglected, ulceration of the vagina. Its use is reserved for the elderly unfit patient or as a temporary measure pending surgery.

Pseudomyxoma peritonei

One of the commonest cystic neoplasms of the ovary is the mucinous cystadenoma. It may be uni- or multi-locular and is filled with a gelatinous substance, mucin. It may reach a *very* large size.

Following rupture of one of these cysts – which may occur spontaneously or at surgery – occasionally, but not always, the cells of the cyst lining implant on the peritoneum and continue to secrete the gelatinous mucin. The peritoneal cavity becomes filled with this mucinous material and bowel adhesions with reactive peritonitis occur. Frequent laparotomies are required to remove as much of the exudate as possible but it inevitably returns and ultimately death occurs from bowel obstruction or cachexia.

Rape

This is defined as 'unlawful sexual intercourse with a woman by force without her consent'. It is a legal diagnosis, not a medical one but doctors may be involved in giving evidence in court. Because the medical examination is a complex one to be sufficient for medico-legal purposes it has been suggested that rape centres should be set up where victims can be taken for detailed assessment.

Points in the examination would include:

1. Examination should be carried out as soon as possible after the incident.
2. A careful history should be obtained if possible.
3. The state of the woman's clothing and general appearance should be noted.
4. The presence of bruising or other injuries noted.
5. The finger nails should be examined for signs of hair – such as would occur after scratching her attacker.
6. Condition of the vulva, hymen and vagina should be recorded.
7. Evidence of staining of clothing with semen or matting of pubic hair should be looked for.
8. Microscopic evidence of semen on clothing or skin, should also be looked for.

Wherever possible the accused male must be examined by a doctor and the presence of bruising, scratch marks, fresh semen, hairs which match the victim's, all looked for.

So far as the management of the victim of rape is concerned, repair of injuries, releasing of haematomata, swabs for infection, antibiotic therapy if appropriate and immediate sedation and pain relief are all involved. In the long term, help must be obtained from social workers and possibly even psychiatrists if the psychological trauma appears profound. Certainly, follow-up of rape victims is desirable both medically and psychologically.

Nursing care

The most important initial action is to ensure that the patient has adequate privacy and the opportunity to talk if she wishes. Analgesia and sedation may be required and will be prescribed accordingly. The nurse should observe any vaginal loss, and any other injury that may be present. Fluids and diet should be encouraged. How much specific nursing care will be required will depend on the extent of the injuries.

The nurse will need to alert the social worker or other counselling agencies as necessary. She will also need to ensure that adequate follow-up is arranged.

Red degeneration

This is a form of degeneration of a fibroid where it has outgrown its blood supply, and breakdown of its central tissues – necrobiosis – occurs. This occurs typically in pregnancy and causes pain.

The only treatment is that required for pain relief.

Sexually transmitted diseases (venereal disease)

This refers to any disease which is transmitted by sexual intercourse. There is a wide variety of such conditions including chancroid, granulosa inguinale and lymphogranuloma venereum but the two most likely to be encountered gynaecologically are gonorrhoea and syphilis. There are now several other prevalent conditions which are sexually transmitted and should by rights be included under the heading. These are chlamydia, genital herpes and of course trichomoniasis (p. 79) and moniliasis (p. 64). AIDS is a modern condition which must also be mentioned in this respect.

Short notes are given on the above conditions. For a fuller description, including complications and problems which may arise, the reader is advised to consult a standard text some of which are listed on page 117.

AIDS

A new disease – acquired immune deficiency syndrome. Mainly described in homosexual men but also found in heterosexuals, drug addicts, Haitians, and haemophiliacs. It can be transferred through affected blood and female partners of affected males.

There is a variety of clinical presentation: pneumonia, fever, a rare sarcomatous tumour (Kaposi sarcoma), fungal or parasitic infections. The death rate from overwhelming infection is high. The basic cause is almost certainly viral and although no specific cure is available as yet research into the cause and the treatment is progressing rapidly.

Chlamydia

Cause   Chlamydia trachomatis, a small Gram-negative intracellular organism requiring special culture medium and fluorescent staining methods for identification. It is probably much more common than realised.

Sites involved   Cervix, urethra, anus. Spread by sexual contact.

Clinical features   Urethritis, cervicitis, pelvic inflammatory disease, trachoma, conjunctivitis.

Treatment   Tetracycline.

Genital herpes

Cause   Herpes virus type 2.

Sites involved   Vulva, vagina, cervix; penis in the male.

Clinical features   Recurrent, exquisitely tender superficial ulceration.

Diagnosis   By special virus culture from active lesions.

Treatment   Apart from local measures the only active anti-viral agent is a drug called acyclovir which can be used locally or systemically.

The fetus has no intrinsic immunity to virus infections and vaginal delivery in the presence of active lesions is dangerous.

Gonorrhoea

Cause   A Gram-negative diplococcus, *Neisseria gonorrhoea.*

Spread   By sexual contact, vaginal, oral and anal.

Sites involved   Tissues not covered by stratified squamous epithelium, e.g. urethra, endocervix, mucosa of mouth or anus.

Clinical features   May be symptomless, or there may be dysuria, frequency, vaginal discharge. Vulvo-vaginitis develops; fever and general malaise; inguinal lymphadenopathy.

Late complications   Pelvic inflammatory disease; joint infections.

Diagnosis   History, examination, Gram stain and culture of urethral and/or endocervical swab.

Treatment   Penicillin. Contacts should be looked for.

Syphilis

Cause   The organism *Treponema pallidum* detected from lesions by dark-ground illumination of fresh specimens of swabs or scrapings. Various serological tests are available, e.g. VDRL tests (Veneral Disease Reference Laboratory).

Spread   A primary ulcer or chancre may appear on the vulva. Incubation is about 1 month during which time the treponema enter the body. The chancre is highly infectious.

Sites involved Vulva, cervix, but anywhere in the body.

Clinical features Usually a pyrexial illness with the appearance of the primary chancre. Lymphadenopathy. Later in the illness mucocutaneous ulcers, skin rashes, warts.

Diagnosis By demonstration of *T. pallidum* in the lesions and positive serology.

Treatment Penicillin or cephaloridine or erythromycin. Reactions to treatment are not uncommon.

Congenital syphilis: A variety of problems can be encountered in the baby of a syphilitic mother. Intra-uterine death or growth retardation, damage to the central nervous system, nephritis, pneumonia, anaemia, skin rashes are some of these conditions.

Sheehan's syndrome

A rare condition following delivery where a severe postpartum haemorrhage has led to necrosis of the anterior lobe of the pituitary gland. Failure to lactate occurs and other endocrine organs then fail to receive their normal stimulus. This leads to:

Adrenal hypofunction with diminution in body hair, lethargy, loss of libido, lack of pigmentation.

Hypothyroidism.

Gonad hypofunction with atrophy of the ovaries and uterus, amenorrhoea, infertility.

Treatment: Replacement therapy must be given.

The condition is rarely seen nowadays where better obstetric management is practised.

Stein-Leventhal syndrome

The older name for polycystic ovarian disease (see p. 68).

Testicular feminisation

In this abnormality of development the chromosome pattern is 46 XY, the gonads are testes but the appearance of the individual is female. The condition is rare and presents more often in a young woman with primary amenorrhoea. Not infrequently inguinal herniae are present in which lie the testes.

The vagina is present but in the form of a blind canal, the uterus is absent and there are rudimentary Fallopian tubes. Because there is a risk of malignant change in the gonads they must be removed after puberty and oestrogen replacement therapy given.

Because no uterus is present, these women cannot have children and, indeed, plastic surgery may be required to form an adequate vagina to enable sexual intercourse to take place.

Thrush infection

Vaginal thrush infection or moniliasis is a frequent cause of discharge and irritation among women.

The cause of the infection is a yeast – *Candida albicans* – which thrives in a warm moist environment such as the vagina provides. Sexual transmission is possible but the source is mainly from the patient's own commensals.

Predisposing conditions are pregnancy, antibiotic therapy and oral contraceptive therapy.

The *appearance* produced is of a red inflamed vulva and vagina with white adherent plaques of the monilial discharge visible on speculum examination. The *diagnosis* is made by laboratory culture.

Treatment is by a variety of antifungal preparations, the commonest being nystatin pessaries.

Toxic shock syndrome

This is a recently described illness predominantly affecting young women, and associated with menstruation and the use of tampons. Most reports have come from the United States of America where a number of deaths were reported. Probably caused by a toxin produced by *Staphylococcus aureus*, the illness is severe and consists of a high fever, skin rashes and hypotension with late involvement of other systems such as the gastro-intestinal system (diarrhoea, vomiting), muscles (myalgia), blood (reduced platelets) and the renal tract (high blood urea).

The condition is rare and further studies are required to elucidate its precise cause.

Trichomoniasis

This vaginal infection is caused by the protozoon *Trichomonas vaginalis* and is a common cause of a thin, yellow foul-smelling discharge causing vaginal soreness and sometimes irritation. Transfer is frequently sexual so that both partners must always be treated..

The *appearance* is of an inflamed vulva and vagina with often copious yellow smelly discharge.

The *diagnosis* can be made by observing the motile flagellated organisms on a fresh wet smear of the discharge or by laboratory culture.

Treatment is by oral metronidazole and must be of both partners.

Urgency of micturition

In this condition the patient feels an irresistible desire to pass urine and unless she can reach a toilet in time may actually be incontinent.

The cause may be instability of the detrusor muscle of the bladder but irritants to the bladder such as infection, calculus or carcinoma must be excluded.

Vaginismus

This is a condition of spasm affecting the sphincter muscles of the vagina and in particular the levator ani muscles. It is a common and important cause of dyspareunia (see p. 43). It may be associated with a tender local lesion of the vulva or vagina but is more often a functional disorder associated with over-anxious frightened women who have had some unpleasant early sexual experience; little or no sexual education, or have a fear of pregnancy, and so on.

The *diagnosis* is usually made by the fact that vaginal examination is either not allowed at all or is carried out with difficulty. Examination under anaesthesia may, rarely, be required to exclude a local lesion and, this being done, *treatment* thereafter is often best done by a psychosexual therapist.

Virilism

Masculinisation of the female as a result of excessive androgen stimulation. It affects muscles (hypertrophy), the larynx, the genitalia and hair distribution.

Causes

1. Ovarian tumour producing androgen (not common).
2. Adrenal tumour.
3. Hypothalamic or pituitary disease.
4. Chromosome abnormality.
5. Drugs, e.g. steroids, androgens.

The cause must be looked for. *Investigations* will include scanning, biochemical tests, laparoscopy. *Treatment*, where possible, is of the cause, e.g. removal of a functioning tumour.

3. Malignant Disease

Malignancy may affect any of the reproductive organs, some being more common than others.

An idea of the relative frequency of gynaecological tumours is shown in Table 3/1. The histological appearance of these tumours varies according to the basic structure of the organ involved.

Table 3/1   The average annual incidence of malignant tumours per million women in the UK

Site	Per million women
Cervix	170
Ovary	150
Endometrium	130
Vulva	30
Vagina	8
Fallopian tube	1

Arrhenoblastoma (see p. 37)

Cervix, carcinoma of (Fig. 3/1)

The cervix is the commonest site for female genital cancer. Some of the recognised aetiological factors are:

Age. 35–60.

Marriage and childbearing. The incidence of the disease in virgins is very low. It appears to be *sexual intercourse* rather than childbearing which is the important factor.

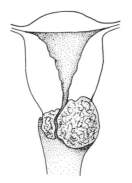

Fig. 3/1 Advanced carcinoma of the cervix

Genetic and racial factors. There is a low risk in Jewesses, high in Africans.

Socio-economic factors. Low socio-economic groups are more at risk.

Cervical irritation and infection. There seems to be a connection between herpes of the cervix and cancer.

Pre-cancerous changes such as dysplasia. This is a state of the epithelium where its growth becomes disordered showing irregularity of size and shape of the cells and their nuclei. This is recognised to be of potential significance.

Types of carcinoma of the cervix

The tumours tend to develop at the squamo-columnar junction; 95 per cent will be squamous cell carcinomas and 5 per cent will arise from the endocervix and are adenocarcinomas.

Adenocarcinoma is nearly always invasive.

Squamous cell carcinoma:

(a) *Carcinoma in situ.* Here the growth is limited to the epithelial layer and is a microscopic rather than a clinical diagnosis.

(b) *Micro-invasive carcinoma.* Here a few cells break through the basement membrane into the stroma.

(c) *Invasive cancer.* The appearance may be of a cauliflower-like growth or ulceration.

Stages

Staging of the disease is as follows:

Stage 0   – carcinoma in situ

Stage I   – invasive but limited to the cervix
    Ia – no visible lesion but invasion to more than 3mm of stroma
    Ib – clinically diagnosed cancer but limited to the cervix
Stage IIa – extending to upper two-thirds of vagina but not to parametrium
    IIb – extending to the parametrium but not reaching the pelvic wall
Stage III – growth extends to
    a – lower third of the vagina
    b – parametrium out to pelvic wall
Stage IV – growth extends to
    a – bladder or rectal mucosa
    b – tissues outside the true pelvis

Clinical features

There may be no symptoms even in invasive carcinoma and the condition may be detected by finding an abnormal smear. The value of routine cervical smears on all women especially those at high risk is unquestionable.

Intermenstrual, postcoital or postmenopausal bleeding may be experienced.

Later in the disease a foul bloodstained discharge develops. Pain is a late feature.

Examination may reveal a normal-looking cervix, or an obvious cauliflower or ulcerative growth.

Management

1. If an abnormal smear is found the following steps are taken depending on the facilities available:
   (a) Colposcopy: This is a technique whereby the cervix can be inspected using a binocular microscope. The epithelium can thereby be inspected directly, abnormal areas identified and precise biopsies taken.
   (b) Cone biopsy of the cervix (see p. 92).
2. If carcinoma in situ is found, the areas may be treated via the colposcope using laser beams to destroy the unhealthy tissue. Cryocautery or electrocautery may also be used. In older women hysterectomy may be carried out.

3. In invasive cancer of the cervix, treatment depends on the staging of the disease and this must be done by appropriate examination (if necessary under anaesthesia) including investigations such as cystoscopy, IVU and sigmoidoscopy.

Then:

In Stages I and II

Extended surgery (Wertheim's hysterectomy) in selected cases. Radiotherapy is the mainstay of treatment.

In Stages III and IV

Radiotherapy. Exenteration operation (see p. 95) may rarely be indicated.

Survival rates (5 year)

Stage I   90 per cent
Stage II   70–75 per cent
Stage III   30–35 per cent
Stage IV   < 10 per cent

Adenocarcinoma is treated as for squamous carcinoma.

Choriocarcinoma

Sometimes referred to as chorioepithelioma, this tumour may follow a hydatidiform mole or a normal pregnancy. It is rare in Western people but more common in Asia.

Irregular bleeding occurs and signs from distant metastases such as bone pain, haemoptysis or pulmonary embolism may develop.

The treatment of choice is chemotherapy using methotrexate. (Generally the patient is either cured of the disease or dies quickly.)

Dysgerminoma

This is a solid ovarian tumour of typical histological appearance consisting of masses of large clear epithelial cells with large nuclei. These tumours are of variable malignancy and are commoner in younger age-groups (under 30).

They are sometimes found in cases of intersex.

Fallopian tube, carcinoma of

This is a rare condition occurring in age-groups 40–60. The presenting symptom is often of recurring heavy watery discharge. Abdominal pain may be present but sometimes the tumour is asymptomatic.

Treatment is by total abdominal hysterectomy and bilateral salpingo–oophorectomy. Radiotherapy or chemotherapy may be given following surgery.

Survival rates are low, between 5 and 25 per cent – probably because of the usual lateness of diagnosis.

Granulosa cell tumours

A solid tumour of the ovary – this produces oestrogen; 5 per cent appear in children leading to precocious puberty, 60 per cent in the childbearing years leading to irregular menstruation and 30 per cent in postmenopausal women leading to postmenopausal bleeding.

They tend to be of low grade malignancy.

Krukenberg tumour

This is a rare secondary tumour of the ovary. The primary growth is usually in the stomach.

Ovary, carcinoma of

Just as there is a confusing variety of benign tumours of the ovary so there is an equally wide range of malignant tumours.

Of all cases of primary carcinoma of the ovary, 80 per cent arise in serous or mucinous cysts; 10 per cent are solid tumours. The remainder may arise from endometrial tissue in the ovary (adeno-carcinoma, adeno-acanthoma, clear-celled carcinoma) or be secondary tumours from primary tumours in breast, stomach or large intestine.

Ovarian cancer occurs in a wide range of age-groups but is commoner after the menopause although not uncommon between 30–40 years. It accounts for a quarter of all genital tract cancer but half the associated deaths. This poor outlook is because the disease is usually silent until quite advanced so diagnosis is often late.

Clinically, presentation is usually by an abdominal mass with or without ascites, abdominal pain, abnormal vaginal bleeding.

Staging and treatment

Stage 1   *Confined to ovary*, either:
- (a)   *Unilateral, intact capsule*. Cystectomy or unilateral oophorectomy and biopsy of the other ovary.
- (b)   *Bilateral, tumour excrescences*. Total abdominal hysterectomy. Bilateral oophorectomy; remove the omentum. Chemotherapy may be given to follow surgery.

Stage 2   *Extension within the pelvis*. As for 1(b) with radiotherapy and/or chemotherapy.

Stage 3   *Extension to abdominal peritoneum*. Surgery followed by chemotherapy. The cisplatinum group of drugs is effective in the treatment of ovarian cancer.

Stage 4   *Extension outside abdomen*. Treatment as for 3 removing as much tumour bulk as possible and following with chemotherapy.

Prognosis depends on stage:

Stage 1 70 per cent 5-year survival

Stage 2 30 per cent 5-year survival

Stage 3 10 per cent 5-year survival

Stage 4 0 per cent 5-year survival

Nursing care

Much of the nursing care for patients with ovarian cancer is aimed at keeping the patient comfortable, particularly in the later stages of the disease. By carefully monitoring the effects of analgesics and anti-emetics the distressing symptoms of pain, nausea and vomiting can be controlled effectively.

ABDOMINAL ASCITES

In the advanced stages of ovarian cancer fluid in the peritoneal cavity (ascites) is a recurring problem necessitating regular paracentesis. As fluid re-collects so breathlessness, pain, nausea and vomiting may increase.

The patient should be nursed in whatever position is most

comfortable for her. Fluids and a light diet should be encouraged; mouth care should be carried out regularly; all pressure areas should be attended to carefully – it may be difficult for the patient to move herself without help; the urinary output should be monitored and bowel movements noted.

Following paracentesis the patient may well be able to return home, albeit briefly. The general practitioner should be kept fully in the picture as he, together with the district nurse and, where there is one, the home terminal care service, will be responsible for the care of the patient.

The patient and her family should be given every opportunity to discuss anything that may be worrying them, be it related to the disease itself or the social and emotional problems resulting from it. The nurse should be prepared to sit and listen to the patient and to help her in whatever way that is appropriate. The social worker, or chaplain may also have a role but may need to be alerted to the need by the nurse.

Uterus, carcinoma of

This is carcinoma of the endometrium. It may be localised or spread diffusely over the surface of the endometrium and be either superficial or invading outwards into the myometrium or downwards into the endocervix. It is a disease of postmenopausal women and usually presents with postmenopausal bleeding. Diagnostic curettage is carried out to establish the diagnosis.

Treatment is by total abdominal hysterectomy and bilateral salpingo-oophorectomy including a cuff of vagina since this is where metastatic deposits may occur. Surgery may be preceded or followed by (more favoured now) radiotherapy.

Prognosis (5-year survival) depends on the stage of the disease:

Stage I	Growth confined to the uterus	80 per cent
Stage II	Growth has extended to the cervix	50 per cent
Stages III and IV	Extension beyond uterus and later into rectum, bladder and other structures outside pelvis	1–2 per cent

Progestogens are useful as an adjunct to treatment.

Sarcoma

This highly malignant but rare tumour arises from muscle or connective tissue, and in gynaecological practice is found either in the uterine wall, in a fibroid or in a fibroma of the vulva.

Treatment is surgical removal, and postoperative radiation may be indicated although it tends to be ineffective in this malignancy. The 5-year survival rate depends upon the stage of the disease and is between 30–45 per cent.

Sarcoma botryoides

This is a rare tumour occurring in childhood. Its appearance may be grapelike or a simple polyp. The prognosis was generally poor but has improved with chemotherapy followed by extensive surgical removal.

Teratoma

This is a germ cell tumour of the ovary and shows a wide histological variety. The benign teratoma or dermoid is commonly filled with sebum and hair and may include bone, cartilage and teeth.

Malignant change may take place in any of the structures.

Vagina, carcinoma of

This is an uncommon malignancy occurring in older women. In the lower part of the vagina tumour cells spread to the inguinal lymph nodes. Carcinoma of the upper vagina behaves like carcinoma of the cervix.

The disease presents itself by bloodstained discharge or frank bleeding.

Radiotherapy is the treatment of choice. The 5-year survival rate depends on the stage of the disease.

Stage 0	In situ carcinoma	100 per cent
Stage I	Confined to vaginal wall	50 per cent
Stage II	Invading tissues deep to vagina	25 per cent
Stages III and IV	Extension to pelvic wall and other viscera	0 per cent

Vulva, carcinoma of (Fig. 3/2)

This is a disease of older women, the commonest site being the labium major followed by the clitoris.

It is usually a squamous cell carcinoma but other rare tumours are melanoma, basal cell carcinoma and sarcoma.

Spread is locally and by the inguinal and femoral lymphatics.

Presentation is often by pruritus, soreness or ulceration.

After establishing the diagnosis by biopsy, the treatment of choice is radical vulvectomy (see p. 109) unless the patient is very frail when only wide excision will be attempted.

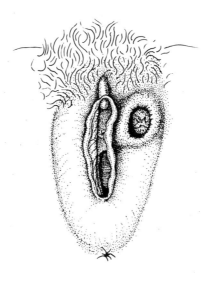

Fig. 3/2 Carcinoma of the vulva

The prognosis depends on spread. There is a 5-year cure rate of 70 per cent if the lymph nodes are not involved; 40 per cent if the superficial nodes are involved; and 20 per cent if deeper pelvic nodes are involved.

Radiotherapy and chemotherapy have no real part to play in treatment.

4. Surgical Procedures

There are several excellent pictorial reference books of gynaeco-logical surgery available (see p. 117). In order to understand a procedure the nurse should not only attend theatre to witness the operation but will find it helpful to consult these textbooks both before and afterwards thereby fixing the broad principles in her mind. Details are unnecessary but basic principles are important for understanding.

In this section a brief outline of such basics for the commoner gynaecological procedures will be given.

Abortion

Although dilatation and curettage (D and C) can be done in the traditional way to effect an abortion, the operation is usually carried out by suction curettage. Hollow metal curettes (Bierer curettes) are available in graded sizes and the one chosen is usually that nearest to the size of the uterus.

After dilatation of the cervix in the usual way, taking care not to overdilate because of the risk of damage to the cervix with subsequent incompetence, the metal curette is attached to suction tubing and a standard pump and the contents of the uterus aspirated out until the cavity is felt to be empty.

Syntocinon is given before the procedure so that the uterus contracts down firmly.

Aldridge sling operation

This is one type of 'sling' procedure used to hitch up the bladder neck in cases of stress incontinence of urine. Strips of fascia from the external oblique aponeurosis are cut and brought down to be sutured together under the urethro-vesical junction.

More modern but similar techniques use materials such as mersilene tape. In all these operations care must be taken not to make the sling too tight. Catheterisation is necessary for some time (a week) after these operations and suitable antibiotics will be required to avoid urinary infection.

Bartholin's cyst: marsupialisation

A cyst of Bartholin's gland may be dissected out and removed complete, *but* an easier and quicker procedure, useful especially if the cyst is infected, is marsupialisation.

An oval shaped piece of skin is excised over the cyst and then an equivalent oval piece of cyst wall. The wall of the now opened cyst is then sutured with interrupted fine catgut sutures to the skin thereby creating an open 'pouch'. The gland itself is thus conserved.

The cavity is packed with ribbon gauze for 24 hours.

Biopsy, of the cervix

With increasing use of colposcopy the procedures to biopsy lesions of the cervix are less used nowadays, but the operation of *cone biopsy* is still employed. The procedure is carried out when a cervical smear shows malignant or dyskaryotic cells and will show histologically whether the lesion is invasive or not, which is important information in the planning of treatment.

Basically, the operation consists in cutting out a cone of tissue from the cervix with a scalpel, beginning the incision circumferentially around the external cervical os. The raw areas left are sutured together with catgut taking care to maintain patency of the cervical canal.

A pack may need to be inserted into the vagina for 24 hours (the operation tends to be haemorrhagic) in which case catheterisation is necessary for 24 hours also.

There is always a risk of immediate and later bleeding in this operation. Theoretically, problems of stenosis or incompetence may arise in a subsequent pregnancy but in practice are rare.

Colpoperineorrhaphy

See repair operations, page 102.

Colposcopy (Fig. 4/1)

This technique is one in which the cervix is visualised through optical instruments. The cellular pattern and vascularity of the epithelium can therefore be studied directly. The colposcope magnifies 10–20 times, the colpomicroscope 100–300 times.

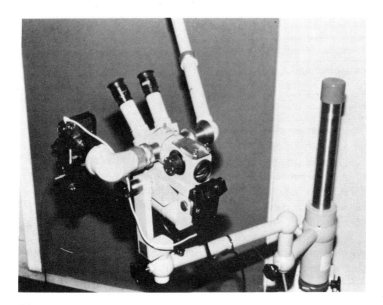

Fig. 4/1 A colposcope

The interpretation of the findings is a matter for an expert in the technique and special clinics are being developed in various centres. It is not yet in use as a routine examination for all women, but is used where an abnormal smear has been found. By means of the procedure, areas of abnormal epithelium can be detected and biopsied directly and benign lesions, such as mild dysplasia, treated with diathermy, cryocautery or laser.

Cryosurgery

Cryocautery of benign lesions of the cervix is a useful and effective procedure because being virtually painless it can be carried out as an outpatient procedure.

Gas (carbon dioxide (CO_2) or nitrous oxide (N_2O)) is passed through a small orifice inside the special cryoprobe and because of its sudden expansion the temperature at the surface of the probe drops to about $-70°C$. Application of the probe to the cervix is usually done for about 2 minutes. The patient will have a watery discharge for about two weeks and should refrain from intercourse during that time. Re-application may be necessary in about 10 per cent of cases 6–10 weeks later.

The procedure is mostly used for cervical erosion, cervicitis or dysplasias under colposcopic control.

Curettage

The operation of dilatation and curettage (D and C) is the commonest minor procedure in gynaecology.

It is most usually carried out for diagnostic purposes – to see the histological appearance of the endometrium. Occasionally it will be a curative procedure, for instance where endometrial polypi are the cause of heavy periods or in the case of retained products of conception.

Under a general anaesthetic and with the patient in the lithotomy position an examination is first carried out to check the pelvic organs and especially to ascertain whether the uterus is anteverted or retroverted. This will indicate in which direction the instruments should be passed in order to avoid perforation of the uterus. The steps are then as follows:

1. The anterior lip of the cervix is grasped with a volsellum forceps.
2. A uterine sound is passed gently into the uterine cavity to measure its length.
3. A polyp forceps or small sponge-holding forceps is then inserted into the cavity and any polypoid tissue grasped and twisted off.
4. A metal curette is then used to curette the uterine cavity systematically – the anterior, posterior and both lateral walls and finally across the fundus. All material thus obtained is sent for

histological examination. The procedure is a minor one and if carried out carefully should have no complications.

Perforation of the uterine wall has been mentioned. If it occurs the procedure should simply be abandoned – the perforation will seal itself – unless there is evidence of malignancy in which case hysterectomy must be carried out. Introduction of infection is always a possibility but with due care and normal precautions this should be avoided.

Nursing care

Following a D and C the nurse should carry out the standard postoperative observations of recording the temperature, respiration rate, pulse rate and blood pressure. In addition she must observe any vaginal loss. Analgesia should be given according to the patient's needs.

Once the patient has recovered from the anaesthetic, and can tolerate them, fluids and a light diet may be restarted.

Diathermy

Electrocautery may be used to treat benign symptomatic lesions of the cervix, such as a cervical erosion. To be effective the procedure needs to be carried out under a general anaesthetic; with the increasing use of cryocautery it tends to be confined to cases who are already having the procedure of dilatation and curettage carried out for other reasons.

Radial linear burns are made on the cervix and as healing of these proceeds the squamous epithelium grows over to cover the ectocervix.

Complications of the procedure are secondary haemorrhage and infection, but with due precautions (e.g. avoidance of intercourse, use of an antibiotic cream) these are relatively rare.

Exenteration, pelvic

This extensive surgery may be indicated in certain cases of pelvic cancer where there is involvement of either the bladder or rectum or both.

Anterior exenteration means removal of the uterus, tubes, ovaries, upper third of vagina, pelvic lymph nodes and the bladder. Re-implantation of the ureters will be necessary either as a ureterocolic implantation or as an ileal bladder.

Posterior exenteration means removal of the genital tract as above plus the rectum. A colostomy will be required.

Total exenteration means removal of the genital tract, the bladder and the rectum. There will be both an ileal bladder and a colostomy.

These procedures carry a high morbidity and where radiotherapy for advanced cancer is a possible alternative it is usually chosen.

Hysterectomy

Removal of the uterus is a common gynaecological procedure. The indications for the operation are variable, ranging from cancer to heavy menstruation either of the dysfunctional type or due to fibroids.

The operation may be carried out by the abdominal route – an *abdominal hysterectomy* – or by the vaginal route – a *vaginal hysterectomy*.

Total hysterectomy refers to the fact that the cervix is also removed; *subtotal*, that it is not removed. Every attempt is made to carry out a total hysterectomy nowadays because of the risk of malignancy in the cervix left in the subtotal procedure. Vaginal hysterectomy is a procedure usually reserved for cases of prolapse. The tubes and ovaries are not normally removed at the vaginal procedure.

If the tubes and ovaries are removed at the abdominal procedure then the full title of the operation is *total abdominal hysterectomy and bilateral salpingo-oophorectomy*.

Psychological preparation for the operation is important in that many women have misinformed and irrational fears about losing the uterus equating it with loss of femininity, the onset of the menopause, growing fat and hairy and so on. The best way to explain it to the worried patient is that the uterus only has two purposes – one to bear children, the other, to menstruate; it does *not* produce hormones and its loss therefore will not cause hormonal changes. In pre-menopausal women it is usual to conserve the ovaries but if they have to be removed hormone implants or hormone replacement therapy will be given.

All this should be explained *before* operation.

The operation (abdominal route)

1. The incision will commonly be a low transverse one, although if the uterus is greatly enlarged by fibroids a paramedian incision may be used.
2. The round ligaments are divided between two clamps thereby opening up the two leaves of the broad ligament.
3. If the ovaries are to be removed a clamp will be placed across the infundibulo-pelvic ligaments thereby dividing the ovarian blood supply. The pedicles are ligated.
4. The loose fold of peritoneum between the uterus and the bladder is now opened so that the bladder can be pushed downwards.
5. The uterine vessels are now clamped and divided by the side of the uterus close to the cervix. The pedicles are sutured.
6. After ensuring that the bladder is pushed downwards clear of the cervix so that the upper vagina becomes visible, curved clamps are placed across the top of the vagina under the cervix and will include not only the vault of the vagina but the cardinal ligaments laterally and the uterosacral ligaments behind, although these latter may be divided separately. Dividing the tissues in these clamps will allow removal of the uterus and cervix.

Complications of the operation may include haemorrhage and damage to other organs (bowel, ureters, bladder) occurring especially where dense adhesions exist due, for example, to endometriosis, pelvic sepsis or cancer.

Late complications are haemorrhage, sepsis and fistulae (urinary or bowel). These last are rare except where malignancy exists.

Other complications are those of any major surgical procedure – ileus (treated by 'drip and suck'), chest or urinary infections and deep venous thrombosis. Nowadays, steps are taken to avoid the last by, for example, the use of early ambulation, the wearing of pressure stockings during and after surgery, small doses of subcutaneous heparin and so on. The incidence of postoperative thombosis has been greatly reduced by these measures. The use of metronidazole, before, during and after pelvic surgery has also significantly reduced the incidence of infection.

The operation of vaginal hysterectomy will not be described separately here. Suffice it to say that the steps are identical, only taken in reverse as the procedure begins with the opening of the vagina.

Variations of the operation of hysterectomy are used where more extensive removal of tissue is required.

A *Wertheim's hysterectomy* is as above but the uterine vessels are divided more laterally to the uterus so that the parametrial tissue on either side can be removed, and the upper third of the vagina is also removed. A pelvic lymph node dissection is also carried out.

The operation is used in certain cases of the earlier stages of cervical cancer.

A similarly radical hysterectomy, but carried out by the vaginal route, is called a Schauta procedure but is not commonly used because of the virtual impossibility of achieving node dissection by this route.

Nursing care

Pre-operatively, the nurse will be involved jointly with the surgeon in ensuring that the woman is adequately prepared and counselled about the operation. Where appropriate the woman's spouse/partner should be included in this preparation.

Postoperatively, the nurse will carry out the standard observations such as recording the temperature, respiration rate, pulse rate and blood pressure. In addition she must observe vaginal loss, and wound drainage.

A catheter may be in situ and the urinary output must be carefully measured and recorded. Similarly, the intravenous infusion needs to be checked regularly. Mouth care should be given as the patient will not be allowed anything by mouth until bowel sounds are heard.

The nurse will observe the patient for signs of restlessness or obvious pain. She must administer analgesia as prescribed and as required thus ensuring a pain-free recovery period for the patient. Breathing exercises and leg exercises, which will have been taught pre-operatively by the physiotherapist, need to be encouraged.

1st postoperative day. The patient can start mobilising gently, for example she can walk round the bed and sit in a chair for a short time. The physiotherapist will continue with breathing exercises and leg exercises, both of which should be encouraged by the nurses. The nurse will continue to record, 4-hourly, the temperature, respiration rate and pulse rate. In addition she will observe and record any wound drainage and the amount of vaginal loss. She will give catheter care and monitor the fluid intake and output. If bowel sounds have returned oral fluids can be started.

2nd postoperative day. Provided bowel sounds have returned satisfactorily oral fluids can be increased with decrease of intravenous fluids. The wound drain may be removed if drainage is minimal. Glycerine suppositories (2) may be given to relieve flatus. Mobilisation can increase; 4-hourly observations should be maintained, and all care given regarding the catheter.

3rd postoperative day, and until discharge. Mobilisation can be increased. Fluids can also be increased and a light diet offered. The wound dressing can be removed and left exposed to the air. The catheter can be removed and urine amounts must be carefully measured; 4-hourly observations should continue, and if the patient is pyrexial a urine specimen and a vaginal swab should be sent for culture.

Sutures and/or clips are removed between the 5th and 7th days. The patient should be shown abdominal exercises by the physiotherapist and taught how to lift correctly.

On discharge the patient should be given written information as well as an oral explanation of what the surgery entailed. She should also be told about how much physical activity she may undertake during the following weeks. If there is a local support group, and if the woman wishes it, she may be given the address.

At all times, both pre- and postoperatively, the nurse should be willing to listen to her patient, to answer questions if she can and to seek advice from others if she cannot.

Hysterotomy

If a pregnancy has to be terminated and the uterus is too large for the procedure to be carried out safely by the vaginal route then an abdominal approach may be used and the uterus emptied through an incision into its cavity. The incision may be made vertically down the middle of the upper segment, or (preferably) transversely through the lower segment after dividing the uterovesical fold of peritoneum which is then closed over the incision line with resultant improvement to the healing process.

The operation of hysterotomy is avoided wherever possible because of its inherent risk for future pregnancies especially where an upper segment incision has been used. Nowadays, the drug prostaglandin may be used instead, either by injecting it into the uterine cavity, or via a catheter inserted through the cervix and advanced alongside the membranes. Prostaglandin induces a miscarriage and open surgery may therefore be avoided.

Laparoscopy (Figs. 4/2, 4/3, 4/4)

This procedure involves passing a long narrow telescope into the peritoneal cavity through a small sub-umbilical incision. To obtain a clear view of the pelvic organs the telescope is attached to a powerful fibre-optic lighting system. In order to insert the telescope safely the peritoneal cavity is first distended with gas (usually nitrous oxide) passed through a special needle.

The value of the procedure is mainly diagnostic in such problems as lower abdominal and pelvic pain and in the investigation of infertility. Surgical procedures such as sterilisation, q.v., can also be carried out.

The procedure is safe in experienced hands but complications can occur; these include damage to a blood vessel with resultant haemorrhage or haematoma formation, and perforation of bowel or bladder.

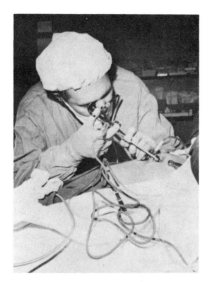

Fig. 4/3 The procedure of laparoscopy

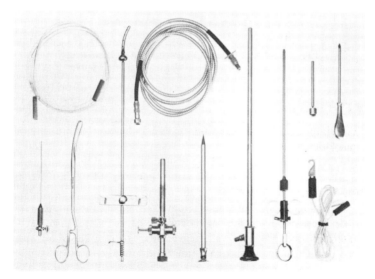

Fig. 4/2 Equipment used for laparoscopy

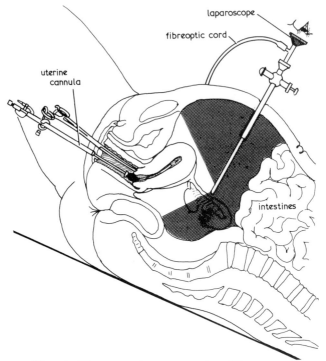

Fig. 4/4 Diagrammatic representation of laparoscopy

Le Fort operation

The simple quick procedure for dealing with a uterine prolapse of major degree is rarely used nowadays. Other operations are more effective and with increasing safety of anaesthesia even the very old can be operated on. Nevertheless the operation still has a place in the management of prolapse in the old and frail.

A rectangular strip of skin is removed from both the anterior and the posterior walls of the vagina and the edges sutured together – anterior wall to posterior wall. The vagina is thereby closed off with two parallel tracts down either side for drainage.

The prime risk is the anaesthetic required, although the procedure could be carried out under local anaesthetic. Haemorrhage and infection are possible but uncommon: recurrence of the prolapse is the main problem, leading as it does to great difficulty in future management.

McDonald suture (also called Shirodkar suture)

In cases of recurrent late abortions the problem may be shown to be an incompetent (open) internal os unable to hold the pregnancy in after 14 weeks.

An insertion of a (braided) nylon suture or tape round the cervix at the approximate level of the internal os will close the os and allow the pregnancy to continue.

The suture is removed at 38 weeks or when labour begins, whichever comes first.

Marshall-Marchetti procedure

This is one of the procedures devised to elevate the bladder neck in cases of stress incontinence. The retropubic space is entered, the urethra exposed and with the help of a Foley catheter in situ the urethro-vesical junction defined. Sutures on either side pick up the vaginal tissue and elevate it to suture it to the periosteum of the back of the pubis.

Problems associated with this operation include retropubic haematoma (a drain should be inserted postoperatively), infection of the site, urinary infection (a catheter is required for some days after surgery), and urinary retention.

Myomectomy

This operation is for removal of fibroids with conservation of the uterus. It is reserved for younger women who wish to preserve their childbearing function. Older women with fibroids are better advised to undergo hysterectomy.

The fibroids are approached through incisions in the *anterior* wall of the uterus if possible (posterior incisions carry the risk of adhesions to bowel). Fibroids have a pseudo-capsule and can be shelled out by the fingers or scalpel handle. Larger ones may be more difficult to remove and a special myomectomy corkscrew can be used. The cavity left after removal of the fibroids is obliterated by deep sutures and the uterine wall then closed.

The complications of this operation are haemorrhage and haematoma formation. Recurrence of fibroids is common.

If the uterine cavity has been opened during the operation this will leave an area of weakness for subsequent pregnancies. In some cases delivery by caesarean section may be indicated rather than risk rupture of such myomectomy scars.

Repair operations

The type of operation used to repair a prolapse of the genital tract depends on the nature and degree of the prolapse.

The following are the common operations employed:

Anterior repair (anterior colporrhaphy)
With a simple cystocele a triangle of skin over the 'bulge' is excised, the bladder dissected up off the skin edges and buttressing or plicating sutures placed in its wall to 'tuck it up'. The skin edges are then closed.

Posterior repair (posterior colpo-perineorrhaphy)
With a rectocele, the posterior wall of the vagina is opened up over the prolapse, redundant skin excised and the skin edges sutured together.

The perineum is re-formed by placing two or three sutures to pull the levator ani muscles together and the remainder repaired as for an episiotomy.

Manchester repair (Fothergill repair)
If there is utero-vaginal prolapse the above procedures are combined with shortening of the cardinal ligaments and amputation of the usually elongated cervix. The shortened ligaments are then sutured together in front of the cervix and the cervical stump re-covered with vaginal skin.

Vaginal hysterectomy
This has already been described and may be combined with an anterior or posterior repair as required (see p. 98).

Repair of an enterocele (see also p. 50)

Like all repairs of true herniae the sac must be identified, excised and ligated and if possible the uterosacral ligaments drawn together to prevent recurrence. This can be done as a separate procedure but is more usually carried out during vaginal hysterectomy.

Nursing care

Following repair of the prolapse and/or a vaginal hysterectomy the nurse will carry out the standard postoperative observations such as recording the temperature, respiration rate, pulse rate and blood pressure. In addition she must observe vaginal loss. A catheter will be in situ and will need to be checked regularly. Similarly, the intravenous infusion must be watched. The nurse will administer analgesics and anti-emetics as prescribed and according to the patient's needs. Mouth care should be given as the patient will not be allowed anything by mouth until bowel sounds are heard. The vaginal pack is usually removed after 24 hours.

1st postoperative day. The patient can start mobilising gently. Deep breathing and leg exercises will be given by the physiotherapist and should be encouraged through the day by the nurses. The nurse will continue to record, 4-hourly, the temperature, respiration rate and pulse rate. The nurse will observe the vaginal loss and carry out catheter care. If bowel sounds are heard, oral fluids can be started.

2nd postoperative day. The intravenous infusion is usually taken down and oral fluids increased, if tolerated, a light diet may be given. The vaginal loss should be checked for colour and odour. Two glycerine suppositories may be given to relieve flatus. If the patient is pyrexial a vaginal swab and urine specimen should be sent for culture and sensitivity. Mobilising should be encouraged.

3rd postoperative day, and until discharge. The patient should be given pelvic floor exercises by the physiotherapist (she will probably have been taught them pre-operatively). She will continue to mobilise and carry out the leg exercises regularly to prevent the development of a deep vein thrombosis. The nurse should encourage the patient to take a well-balanced diet, and plenty of fluids to promote bowel action.

Before discharge the patient should be given written information about the operation performed. In addition she should be given clear advice (if necessary this should be written as well) concerning the amount and type of physical activity allowed. Correct lifting should be taught before the patient returns home.

Sterilisation

There are several methods of sterilising the female. Before any surgery is done adequate counselling must be given. Both female and male parties should, ideally, be agreeable and seeking the operation; they should understand its finality and its failure rate.

Theoretically the operation is reversible but at the present time the procedure should not be undertaken with the idea that it can be undone if required in the future. The failure rate is small (a round figure of 1 in 1000 is useful to remember) but significant and must be understood by the couple to avoid medico-legal complications later.

The operations

LAPAROSCOPIC METHODS

After insertion of the laparoscope and visualisation of the tubes these are picked up by special long forceps passed through a separate side cannula and either destroyed by diathermy (not popular now because of the risk of burns to, for example, the bowel), clipped or banded. The latter involves drawing a loop of tube through a small silastic ring; clips are of several varieties, the most commonly used being the Hulka-Clemens clip or the Filshie clips.

Complications are those of laparoscopy (see p. 100).

LAPAROTOMY

Through a very small incision (mini-laparotomy) the tubes are brought to the surface and either clipped or clamped and divided.

At a more formal laparotomy a Pomeroy procedure may be carried out where a loop of tube is ligated at its base with catgut and the loop excised. A variation of this is to excise a portion of the tube and bury the ends in the broad ligament.

This open method is used at the time of other surgery, such as caesarean section.

OTHER METHODS

Culdoscopy. Access to the tubes is through the posterior fornix. Once located they are dealt with as above.

Salpingectomy. Removal of the entire tube on each side is certainly a more complete method of sterilisation and may be done at the time of laparotomy.

Hysteroscopy. A hysteroscope is a fibreoptic instrument used to inspect the interior of the uterine cavity. Through it the tubal openings can be visualised and closed by chemicals, cautery or plugs. This method is not yet in general use.

Hysterectomy. Removal of the uterus itself is an effective method of sterilisation and in the presence of problems such as fibroids, intractable menorrhagia, and so on, should be recommended as the method of choice in a couple seeking sterilisation.

Trachelorrhaphy

This operation consists of excising the torn and unhealthy section of a cervix and then refashioning the cervix. It is used only for benign conditions and, in fact, is rarely indicated.

Tubal surgery

Operations on the tubes are carried out in cases of infertility where the primary problem is tubal blockage of one kind or another. The technique of microsurgery has greatly improved results but in general the more extensive the blockage and therefore the more elaborate the surgery required the less successful is the outcome.

The operations

SALPINGOLYSIS

In the simplest cases it may be possible to relieve tubal obstruction merely by dividing peri-tubal adhesions and freeing the tube.

SALPINGOSTOMY

Previous investigations will have demonstrated that the blockage exists at the fimbrial end of the tube and the appearance at laparotomy is of a rounded smooth 'clubbed' fimbrial end.

The procedure consists of freeing the end of the tube, slitting it open and turning back the end rather like the cuff of a sleeve so as to maintain patency. Sometimes a plastic splint is passed along the tube into the uterus, and sutured to the ampullary end where it is left for a week or two to help maintain patency.

A variation of this operation is to use a thimble-shaped plastic device with an internal 'tongue' which is stitched over the opened end of the tube, the tongue being inserted into the lumen of the tube. In this way patency is maintained during healing. The disadvantage of this device – the Rock-Mulligan Hood – is that it requires a further laparotomy 8 to 10 weeks later for its removal.

UTERO-TUBAL IMPLANTATION

This procedure is used where there is blockage at the cornual end of the tube. This section of the tube is excised and the outer patent portion re-implanted into the uterus. The use of polythene rods as splints to maintain patency is necessary and they are removed from the uterine cavity by the vaginal approach after about 2 to 3 months.

Varying success rates are reported for these operations: salpingolysis 30 to 40 per cent; for salpingostomy 10 to 15 per cent and for tubal implantation 10 to 20 per cent.

Where surgery seems impractical because of the severity of pelvic disease, in vitro fertilisation is now being used increasingly. Here ova are removed from ripe follicles, using the laparoscope, and are then fertilised in vitro by the husband's sperm; when this is successfully achieved the fertilised egg is placed back into the mother's uterine cavity where the endometrium has been 'primed' by progesterone. With increasing use of this technique, and therefore increasing success, the need for difficult surgery on severely damaged tubes will diminish.

Ventrosuspension

This operation aims to swing the uterus forward into a position of anteversion and fix it in that position.

The procedure used to be carried out quite commonly but nowadays it is realised that a retroverted uterus does not cause serious problems and that surgery is not necessary. Nevertheless there are occasions when it is felt to be justifiable. For instance, if a woman suffers from endometriosis with a fixed retroversion and perhaps an ovary prolapsed into the pouch of Douglas, she is likely to suffer from deep dyspareunia and added to the treatment of the endometriosis a ventrosuspension will relieve the symptoms.

The operation is usually carried out by plicating the round ligaments with a non-absorbable material such as black silk and suturing them to the rectus sheath on either side. Simple plication of the round ligaments only is sometimes done but this is not so effective.

Vulvectomy (Fig. 4/5)

This operation may be either simple or radical. The simple procedure removes the skin and deeper tissues of the vulva; the radical procedure involves a much wider excision of skin, deep tissue and lymph nodes of groins and femoral triangles. The diagrams of the incisions for these two procedures demonstrate their extent.

Simple vulvectomy is carried out for benign lesions of the vulva such as intractable dysplasias. The radical operation is carried out for malignant disease of the vulva.

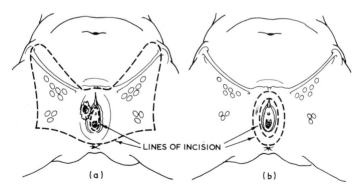

Fig. 4/5 Incisions for vulvectomy: (a) radical; (b) simple

Nursing care

The nurse will be involved with explanation to the patient of the extent of the operation and the possible after-effects. While the doctor will explain clinical matters to the patient it is the nurse who will almost certainly have to answer questions, allay worries and to offer reassurance not only to the woman but to her partner also. This will commence pre-operatively and will certainly continue postoperatively.

Postoperative nursing care will include the standard observations of temperature, respiration rate, pulse rate and blood pressure. The catheter will require regular attention as will any intravenous infusions which may be in situ. Fluid intake and output must be carefully monitored and recorded. The wound will require constant care and observation.

Wound care. A non-adherent dressing is applied in theatre and left, usually for 24 hours. Thereafter twice daily dressings will be required, and if they are heavily soiled will need re-applying more frequently. The wound should be cleaned with half-strength eusol and Debrisan may be applied to keep the wound clean and to encourage granulation. A Silastic Foam dressing may be used as an alternative.

Diet. Because the wound may be large (radical vulvectomy) and, until healing starts, may have almost continuous serous loss, a high protein diet with plently of fluids should be encouraged.

Sutures. These are usually removed about the 14th day.

Urinary catheter. This will remain in place until the wound area is small and is healing well. Catheter care should be given each time the wound is dressed. As the patient becomes more mobile, bathing and the use of a bidet can be encouraged.

Mobilisation. Breathing exercises and leg exercises should be taught pre-operatively and encouraged postoperatively. Mobilisation will be gradual according to the patient's general condition

5. Hormones and Related Drugs

The sex hormones play a large part in gynaecological management. Their use, for instance, in the contraceptive pill is widely known, but other uses are made of them and these will be mentioned here. Related drugs are also described.

Androgens

An androgen is a substance which has the capacity to produce masculinity. They are therefore the male sex hormones but are produced in the female, the most important being *testosterone*. The chief source is the adrenal cortex.

Action of androgens in the female
1. Atrophy of uterus, vagina, vulva, breasts.
2. Arrest of the ovarian cycle.
3. Physiologically responsible for axillary and pubic hair. Excess will lead to virilisation.

Uses in gynaecology
1. In sexual frigidity androgens appear to have a beneficial affect. Testosterone may be given in implant form along with oestrogen.
2. In problems of metabolism they may be used for their anabolic effect, e.g. in anorexia nervosa.

The chief undesirable side-effect is virilisation of the female.

Bromocriptine

One of the pathological causes of an excess production of the hormone prolactin from the pituitary is deficiency of the substance dopamine. The drug bromocriptine is a dopamine agonist and therefore reduces the level of prolactin.

Hyperprolactinaemia is seen with adenomas (or microadenomas) of the anterior pituitary and leads to amenorrhoea and inappropriate lactation or galactorrhoea. Bromocriptine will reduce the prolactin level leading to restoration of periods and suppression of lactation. Fertility is restored where this has been an associated problem, and the pituitary adenoma appears to regress.

Bromocriptine is also used in benign breast disease and it can be used for suppression of lactation after childbirth.

Chorionic gonadotrophins

See gonadotrophins, page 113.

Clomiphene citrate

This is an anti-oestrogen substance blocking the inhibitory action of oestrogen on the hypothalamic-pituitary system and therefore causing release of gonadotrophins.

It is therefore of value where there is failure of ovulation and is of considerable value in the management of anovulatory infertility.

The dosage given to begin with is 50mg daily for 5 days starting on the third day of menstruation, or empirically if there is associated amenorrhoea. Its effect can be monitored by the use of a temperature chart or by measuring the serum level of progesterone on about day 19 of the cycle.

Clomiphene induces ovulation in about 70 per cent of cases but the pregnancy rate is about half that figure.

There is a higher incidence of twins and an abortion rate as high as 25 per cent is reported.

Cyproterone acetate

This is an anti-androgen and has important clinical application in the management of hirsutism and acne in women.

Danazol

This is a synthetic steroid which lowers the levels of FSH and LH. This anti-gonadotrophic action is strong enough to suppress ovulation and menstruation.

Its main use is in the treatment of endometriosis but it is also of value in benign breast disease and menorrhagia. It is given in tablet form and the average dosage is between 200 and 600mg daily in divided doses.

Gonadotrophins

A combination of FSH and LH will have a direct effect on the ovaries inducing ovulation. In practice two sources are required, one for FSH and the other for LH.

The urine of postmenopausal women contains relatively large amounts of FSH. This provides the commercial source of Human Menopausal Gonadotrophin (HMG) which provides the main source of FSH used for therapy in Europe and the USA.

Human chorionic gonadotrophin (HCG) has the same properties as LH and is prepared from the urine of pregnant women.

These two agents are powerful inducers of ovulation and their use must be monitored most carefully if overstimulation of the ovaries is not to occur. Ovulation results in a high proportion of cases but again the pregnancy rate is lower, although figures as high as 90 per cent are quoted. There is a high incidence of multiple pregnancies with the resultant risk of abortion or premature labour.

Injectable contraceptive

Intramuscular injections of a depot progestogen, such as medroxy-progesterone acetate (Depo-Provera) 150mg given every 3 months will provide quite effective contraception. Side-effects are few and it is a suitable method for Third World countries or where women are unreliable pill takers and have problems with IUCDs.

Oestrogens

These are the 'chief' female hormones and as oestradiol, oestriol and oestrone are synthesised mainly in the ovaries. Some is produced from the adrenal cortex and the human placenta.

They are metabolised in the liver. Oestradiol and oestrone are the active oestrogens and are used therapeutically.

Oestrogens are used in all age-groups and for a variety of conditions. Because of their relationship with thrombosis their use and dosage systemically must be carefully controlled.

Examples of use of oestrogens:

Vulvo-vaginitis of infancy and children (cream form).

Control of menstruation in reproductive age-groups (combined with a progestogen).

Contraception (in combination with a progestogen).

Hormone replacement therapy (in the postmenopausal age-groups).

Progesterone

This 'other' female hormone is secreted by the corpus luteum, the placenta and the adrenal cortex. The synthetic products are called progestogens, and although natural progesterone is now available it is the synthetic products which are mostly used. Progesterone is metabolised by the liver.

Like oestrogens, progestogens are used in a variety of conditions and age-groups:

Menstrual regulation: alone or in combination with oestrogen.

Contraception: alone, as in the so-called 'mini-pill', or in combination with oestrogen.

As part of hormone replacement in the menopausal age-groups.

As an adjunct to treatment of carcinoma of the endometrium.

Prolactin

A hormone produced by the anterior pituitary especially in pregnancy where its chief role is in the initiation of lactation. A tumour (adenoma) of the anterior pituitary may raise the level of prolactin in the non-pregnant woman. Hyperprolactinaemia results in associated amenorrhoea, galactorrhoea (inappropriate lactation) and infertility. The drug bromocriptine lowers the level of prolactin and permits fertility. For larger adenomata, surgical removal or radiotherapy may be required.

Prostaglandins

These are unsaturated fatty acids produced by all mammalian cells and first identified in human seminal fluid. They have the capacity to stimulate smooth muscle. Those chiefly used in obstetrics and gynaecology are prostaglandin E_2 (PGE_2) and prostaglandin $F_{2\alpha}$ ($PGF_{2\alpha}$).

Their uses are mainly in preparation of the cervix (ripening) for induction of labour, or in induction of mid-trimester abortion (given either extra-amniotically by a catheter inserted through the cervix, or injected trans-abdominally directly into the uterine cavity).

Prostaglandins may play some part in the aetiology of dysmenorrhoea and the use of prostaglandin antagonists such as mefenamic acid has proved successful in the treatment of this condition.

Syntocinon

This is a synthetic oxytocin, the latter being a hormone released by the posterior pituitary.

It stimulates uterine muscle and is therefore used in induction of labour, enhancement of labour, postpartum haemorrhage, and to control the bleeding of abortion.

Testosterone

This is the more important of a group of hormones causing masculinisation and collectively called androgens. The chief source in the female is the adrenal gland. It is metabolised in the liver.

Excess of testosterone in the female such as may arise with adrenal or some ovarian tumours causes hirsutism and other signs of virilisation.

Therapeutically testosterone may be of some value in the treatment of sexual frigidity especially in the postmenopausal woman.

Further Reading

Anderson, M. (rev.) (1979). *The Anatomy and Physiology of Obstetrics: a short textbook for students and midwives*, 6th edition. Faber and Faber, London.

Anderson, M. (1983). *The Menopause*. Faber and Faber, London.

Bailey, R. E. and Grayshon, J. (1983). *Obstetric and Gynaecological Nursing*, 3rd edition. Bailliere Tindall, London.

Barnes, J. (1983). *Lecture Notes on Gynaecology*, 4th edition. Blackwell Scientific Publications Limited, Oxford.

Fox, H. and Buckley, C. H. (1983). *An Atlas of Gynaecological Pathology*, MTP Press, Lancaster.

Fream, W. C. (1979). *Notes on Gynaecological Nursing*. Churchill Livingstone, Edinburgh.

Lees, D. H. and Singer, A. *A Colour Atlas of Gynaecological Surgery*, six volumes. Wolfe Medical and Scientific Publications, London.

Llewellyn-Jones, D. (1986). *Fundamentals of Obstetrics and Gynaecology*, 4th edition: volume 1 *Obstetrics*, volume 2 *Gynaecology*. Faber and Faber, London.

Llewellyn-Jones, D. (1986). *Everywoman: A Gynaecological Guide for Life*, 4th edition. Faber and Faber, London.

Llewellyn-Jones, D. (1985). *Herpes, AIDS and Other Sexually Transmitted Diseases*. Faber and Faber, London.

McCormack, W. M. (ed.) (1982). *Diagnosis and Treatment of Sexually Transmitted Diseases*. John Wright and Sons Limited, Bristol.

Mandelstam, D. (ed.) (1980). *Incontinence and its Management*. Croom Helm, London.

Reynolds, M. (1984). *Gynaecological Nursing*. Blackwell Scientific Publications Limited, Oxford.

Shorthouse, M. and Brush, M. (eds.) (1981). *Gynaecology in Nursing Practice*. Bailliere Tindall, London.

Tiffany, R. (ed.) (1978). *Cancer Nursing – Medical*. Faber and Faber, London.

Tiffany, R. (ed.) (1979). *Cancer Nursing – Radiotherapy*. Faber and Faber, London.

Tiffany, R. (ed.) (1980). *Cancer Nursing – Surgical*. Faber and Faber, London.

Tindall, V. R. (1981). *A Colour Atlas of Clinical Gynaecology*. Wolfe Medical and Scientific Publications, London.

Useful Organisations

There are a number of self-help groups throughout the United Kingdom. The following addresses are those of the main agency who would be able to direct enquirers to the nearest group to their home.

The Patients Association
Room 33, 18 Charing Cross Road
London WC2H 0HR   01–240 0671

This association publishes a handbook *Self-Help and the Patient*.

London Rape Crisis Centre
PO Box 69, London WC1X 9NJ   01–837 1600

The address of such a centre in each locality will be found in the area telephone directories. There are centres in all major towns and cities.

Endometriosis Self-Help Group
65 Holmdene Avenue
Herne Hill, London SE24 9LD   01–737 4764

Hysterectomy Support Group
Ravendell, Warren Way
Lower Heswall, Wirral
Merseyside L60 9HU   051–342 3167

National Association for Premenstrual Tension
c/o 23 Upper Park Road
Kingston-upon-Thames, Surrey KT2 5LB

Index